READING RESEARCH

How to make research more approachable

Second Edition

Margaret E Ogier

RGN, RM, DipN, RNT, BSc, PhD, C Psychol

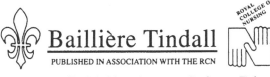

Baillière Tindall

PUBLISHED IN ASSOCIATION WITH THE RCN

London Philadelphia Toronto Sydney Tokyo

Baillière Tindall
An imprint of Harcourt Publishers Limited

 is a registered trademark of Harcourt Publishers Limited

© 1998 Baillière Tindall
© 1999 Harcourt Publishers Limited

This book is printed on acid-free paper

First published 1989
Reprinted 1999

A catalogue record for this book is available from the British Library

ISBN 0-7020-2338-8

Typeset by Phoenix Photosetting, Chatham, Kent
Printed and bound in Great Britain by Bell and Bain Ltd, Glasgow

Key Words

- Understanding research
- Evidence-based practice
- Information technology
- Nursing
- Literature search

Q
APP

READING RESEARCH

How to make research more approachable

610. 73072

OGI

Contents

Acknowledgements

Thanks are due to many people who have contributed their knowledge, expertise and enthusiasm at various points from the inception to publication of this booklet:
Without the good will and hard work of many trained nurses, from enrolled to senior nurse managers and educators, who have attended the Research Workshops upon which this booklet is based the ideas and concepts would not have evolved.

To Caroline Foster-Dean, the late Harry Gallagher, Heather Gough, and Pierre Herve thanks for reading the preliminary manuscript, commenting and encouraging me to offer the booklet for publication.

To the nurse researchers who reviewed the manuscript and gave of their time and expertise to refine and improve the original concepts I owe a large debt of gratitude.

For the clarity of expression, enthusiasm and support I sincerely thank Richenda Milton-Thompson. My thanks go, too, to Michael Dixon for advice on the Results section.

If it had not been for Rosemary Morris, Carrie Walker and the staff at Scutari publishers showing patience and faith in this booklet it would not have reached this stage. To you all many thanks.

Many thanks to you the nurses who have read and used the first edition and encouraged the writing of a second edition.

I appreciate the advice and expertise of the reviewers and nurse researchers who have willingly shared their work.

Without the help of several librarians such as those at the Royal College of Nursing and Valerie Rowland and Ruth Smale of the Nurse Education Library, Guernsey who with patience and good humour found the most obscure journal articles and followed up references for me, writing this second edition would have been impossible.

Thanks to Jacqui Curthoys of Baillière Tindall for her support, enthusiasm and bright ideas.

Special thanks to my husband John for his support in many different ways and his patience while I disappeared under piles of paper and books.

Without the efforts of all mentioned above the material would not have appeared in the form it is today. While every effort has been taken to be accurate while being brief, as author, I accept the responsibility for any weakness or inaccuracy.

1
Introduction: how to use this book

Key words:
- Informed practice
- Evidence-based practice
- Research-based profession

'Research? That's something people do in university departments or laboratories isn't it? It doesn't have much to do with real life does it? Isn't it something nurses do if they feel they are not very good at proper bedside care?'

This is the opening remark from the first edition written in 1989. For a few readers the sentiments may still be true, but many more nurses are aware of the key role of research or at least acknowledge the importance of research findings in informing their practice. This edition retains the original aim from the first edition: to make reading research reports a feasible and enjoyable task. If you can find a way of interpreting and understanding research then you will be working towards evidence-based practice. You should develop an awareness of **G** research findings together with critical reading skills so that you can be selective in choosing the most appropriate findings and, where necessary, seek further support for some findings and discard others on an informed basis. With the drive to make nursing a research-based profession there is a danger that rather **G** than rejecting research, as in the opening quotation, nurses may feel compelled to adopt a particular piece of research just because it *is* research, without giving the results and their implications due critical, knowledgeable scrutiny.

This book is intended as a guide, but also as a stimulus for further reading and appreciation of nursing research. It is written from my experience of working with qualified nurses who have not encountered research reports previously, and is not intended to belittle what you already know. However, I assume that the nurse education programme you followed did not leave you feeling competent and/or confident to scrutinize research findings; alternatively, you may be embarking on a programme of education. This book will help you get started.

As the text is designed to be readable and concise, it is inevitable that some terms, ideas and issues will not be mentioned. There are several books on the research process, some more readable than others, some more detailed than others. This book does not aim to compete with them, but rather gives you a 'jumping-off point' from which to tackle them. Indeed you are advised to have access to at least one of them. Above all, this text *does not prepare you to do research*. Indeed, Mead (1996) highlights the dangers of students and nurses attempting small-scale research projects as part of their educational programme.

How to use this book

The key words at the start of this introduction give the reader a hint of the main topics included in the chapter. Each chapter has key words and these are in bold type in the text.

Icons in the margin indicate where there is further reading (▨), reference to a term in the Glossary (**G**➤) or a cross-reference.

In order to help explain a point, brief boxed examples are included.

Short self-assessment questions are included at various points and are indicated by ▨ in the margin.

The next chapter considers the reasons for doing research. Chapter 3 discusses how to find research reports. After that, each chapter follows the order of a research report, addressing each section in turn, i.e. literature review, method, results, etc.

2
Why bother about research?

Key words:
- Critical reading
- Research application
- Nursing excellence
- Knowledge

Before we begin, let us go back to a thorny question: why bother about nursing research at all? This chapter briefly considers professional, clinical and personal reasons why the understanding and application of nursing research findings is important.

Professional development

Perhaps a good place to start is with a quotation:

> 'When nurses' sensitivity to human needs (their intuition) is joined with the ability to find and use expert opinion, with the ability to find reported research and apply it to their practice, and when they themselves use the scientific method of investigation, there is no limit to the influence they might have on health care worldwide.' (Henderson, 1987)

This ideal appears to have been incorporated into the modern philosophy of nursing and health care. It is in evidence in three recent reports highlighted by the Chief Nurse at the Department of Health in September 1996. She writes that there is enthusiasm and commitment to health-care research but also there is need for the development of critical analysis skills (Moores, 1996). The Culyer Report (Department of Health, 1994) emphasizes the need for evidence-based practice and the need to evaluate the impact of different interventions. Similar ideas are stated in the *Research and Development Strategy for the National Health Service in Scotland* (Scottish Office Home and Health Department, 1993). In July 1996 a report on a three-year investigation into the implementation of research findings, identifying barriers, expectations, achievements and opportunities for the future was published by the Foundation of Nursing Studies (1996). As well as advocating more nursing research, these reports all discuss the need to disseminate research findings so that they will be accessible to staff in clinical practice, management and education. Finally, each report highlights the need to increase the skills of practitioners in **critical reading** and appraising research. It is hoped that this book will enable you eventually to provide research-based care.

The **excellence** and commitment demanded of nurses is reinforced by the United Kingdom Central Council for Nursing, Midwifery and Health Visiting (1992) Code of Professional Conduct, which exhorts all nurses, midwives and health visitors to:

> 'Act always in such a manner as to promote and safeguard the interest and wellbeing of patients and clients ... [and] maintain and improve your professional knowledge and competence.'

Nurses who are content to learn by rote and continue to perform a particular procedure because 'it has always been done that way' on their ward will never approach this level of excellence. Indeed, the care they deliver may be actually harmful and bad.

Clinical development

One subject where the importance of research findings can be easily seen is in the care of pressure areas. There has been an enormous amount of research conducted on this topic since the pioneering work of Doreen Norton in 1962 (Norton et al., 1962). Unfortunately, however, there are still wards and hospitals throughout the country where research is considered to be something that has no relation to clinical nursing. Practices such as the use of air rings to relieve pressure are still common (Deacon, 1986), and ideas on treatments are as varied as the individual nurses (Bromley, 1986) Many rituals still continue even though they have been shown to be harmful.

Hulland (1985), who studied nurses' actions and beliefs in relation to pressure sore prophylaxis and treatment, concludes that nurses are well disposed to the Norton Score and can identify factors that predispose a patient to develop pressure sores but that they do not follow through with the required care. She suggests that this is due to the nurses' limited lack of in-depth knowledge and experience, which results in an adherence to ritual and routine that predetermines the care a patient receives. However, Isles (1986) describes his determined efforts to educate and support the nursing staff in his area in order to reduce and prevent pressure sores effectively. He documents the decrease in the incidence and severity of sores after his sustained efforts to encourage nurses to be better informed and to *use* their knowledge of research findings.

Carrying out a computer-based literature search (CINAHL) in order to update the references for this edition, I found 18 journal articles in 1995 related to pressure areas and the variety of methods to relieve pressure. So there is plenty of research going on and it is being reported in accessible journals held in most local nurse libraries. However, it is doubtful that research findings are being widely used to inform everyday practice, as indicated in the report *Strategy for Research in Nursing, Midwifery and Health Visiting* (Department of Health, 1993):

see Chapter 3

'There is a need to create a climate where research is respected and used in practice. Managers, practitioners and educators should all be a part of this process. There is also a clear role for both purchaser and providers.' (Annexe 3.2.3)

Let us consider another area, the psychological aspects of care. How much do we depersonalize patients and staff? One study found that patients' anxiety on admission was reduced when the nurses were friendly and called the patients by their name (Franklin, 1974). In my own study (Ogier, 1982), student nurses felt happier and thought they had learnt more in wards where other staff recognized them as individuals, as Mary or David and not just another student. The ability to address another person by name does not require a complex educational programme; rather it is a basic courtesy that research has shown to be missing in many instances. By increased sensitivity to others' needs, patient care and staff morale can be inexpensively improved. This is not to say that training in communication and interpersonal skills should not be given and the need for these have been highlighted by several researchers (e.g. Powell, 1982; Gott, 1984).

One community health council carried out a year-long survey to monitor the quality of information-giving, with a sample of 1500 patients discharged from acute hospitals. The results show a generally high level of satisfaction with the information related to surgical and technical procedures. Less technical aspects of care, such as reasons for bed rest, were less well explained. Some patients found staff insensitive in the way that they conveyed upsetting or disappointing news (Cortis and Lacey, 1996).

At a deeper level of interpersonal understanding, Twomey (1987) encourages us to look more closely at the patients' needs and not to jump to conclusions as to what we think they need. In considering Ann Tait's in-depth study of one patient, Twomey looks at the issues surrounding the woman who undergoes mastectomy. She identifies the concerns of many women as being not only with the mutilation but also with the implications of having cancer. Faulkner (1984), amongst others, looked at the incidence of clinical depression in women who had mastectomies and the role of the nurse in helping patients adjust to the trauma. In an effort to compensate for some of these weaknesses, Edmonstone (1996) reports on an initiative by the Scottish Department of Health to carry out a research programme that would empower nurses working with cancer patients.

All this may sound very academic, but just think for a moment. If someone close to you had just undergone a traumatic operation, you would want every opportunity to be taken to help them adjust to a new body image without further distress. If you think about it as a caring nurse rather than as a concerned relative you would probably wish the same. As a nurse, familiarity with research findings in a number of studies, including those cited here, will make it easier for you to achieve this.

Personal development

Research studies also look at nursing and nurses, as well as patients. For instance, research into the influences on nursing staff's perception of stress in the operating theatre has shown that difficulties with the organization of staff meal breaks produces highly significant stress levels (Astbury, 1988). Spouse (1990) highlights the stress on both the qualified nurse and the student as they try to match service and educational needs within the clinical area.

'Knowledge is power' is a very old saying. What familiarity with research findings does is to broaden your **knowledge** and give you ammunition to use in your fight for better care, better opportunities and better quality of life for your patients. Familiarity with research findings can help you to avoid complications that are costly in terms of money and human suffering. Such familiarity may also broaden your knowledge in such a way as to enable you to make conditions better and learning easier for you and your staff. The secret lies in knowing how to access research findings, to evaluate research reports and how to implement appropriate findings, thereby beginning to bridge the theory–practice gap.

3
How to find what you need to read

Key words:
- Key words
- Synonyms
- Information technology
  Database
  MEDLINE

  CINAHL
  BNI
  Internet/Web site
- Abstracting journals

If you have found a research report you want to read or if you have been given a piece of research to read then you are ready to start. If not, you may like to 'browse' through some nursing journals and identify research reports to whet your appetite.

There are so many nursing journals it is difficult to know where to start, so in the Further reading section I have indicated some that contain more research reports than others. Stodulski (1995) carried out a study of UK nursing journals and rated the journals for levels of research content; the following are those rated as containing high levels of research:

- *Intensive and Critical Care Nursing*
- *International Journal of Nursing Studies*
- *Journal of Advanced Nursing*
- *Midwifery*
- *Nurse Education Today*
- *Nurse Researcher.*

These might be a starting point to identify a journal with a high research content if you just want to familiarize yourself with the type of relevant article.

It is important to note that in the future more and more journals are likely to increase their research content as the drive for evidence-based practice and a research-based profession continues.

Starting point

First, clarify the topic. If you have not been given a particular issue to read about but there is a particular question you would like to investigate, the first step is to write it out in your own words.

> The question I wanted to answer when I had the opportunity to carry out some research was: 'What is it about some ward sisters that they make student nurses feel they have learnt something, while with other sisters students are left with the feeling that they have just survived an obstacle course?' (I know this book is not about you carrying out research but the starting point is the same. In order to research into anything, you have to find out what is already known; in other words you have to carry out a literature search to look for research studies already carried out in that area.)

It is useful to share and discuss your ideas with colleagues and friends. Rethink your question in the light of the discussions that arise from sharing it. It is wise to do this on several occasions as each time you explain your ideas you are clarifying and refining them. It may be particularly helpful to find a non-nurse willing to listen to your ideas. A lay person is likely to question aspects that we as nurses take for granted or as unchallenged facts.

Now you may need, or like, to rewrite your original idea. My final research question was: 'What is it about a ward sister's leadership style and verbal interaction with nurse learners that affects their (the student's) learning?' (Ogier, 1982).

 Next underline the **key words** (there should be no more than six of these). From the example above, the key words might be 'sister' and 'learning'.

 List the key words and beside each write as many **synonyms** or words that you think mean the same or are closely similar:

- Sister   charge nurse, head nurse
- Learning   studying, teaching, understanding.

What is the point of this exercise? If you are like me you are no doubt short of time and rush into the library 15 minutes before it is due to close. By the time you have caught your breath and decided what it is you want, you are being asked to leave. However, if you have spent some time thinking through your ideas before you rush into the library, you will be able to make a coherent request to the librarian who will be much better able to help you. Or, if you make your own search, you

Baillière Tindall

24–28 Oval Road
London, NW1 7DX

The Curtis Center
Independence Square West
Philadelphia, PA 19106–3399, USA

Harcourt Brace & Company
55 Horner Avenue
Toronto, Ontario, M8Z 4X6, Canada

Harcourt Brace & Company, Australia
30–52 Smidmore Street
Marrickville
NSW 2204, Australia

Harcourt Brace & Company, Japan
Ichibancho Central Building
22-1 Ichibancho
Chiyoda-ku, Tokyo 102, Japan

First published 1989

A catalogue record for this book is available from the British Library

ISBN 0-7020-2338-8

Typeset by Phoenix Photosetting, Chatham, Kent
Printed and bound in Great Britain by Bell and Bain Ltd, Glasgow

Key Words

- Understanding research
- Evidence-based practice
- Information technology
- Nursing
- Literature search

Figure 3.1   Sample bibliographic page.

will at least know where to start. I suggest you put alternatives next to your key words because your first word may draw a blank in the subject index. 'Sister' is not likely to draw a blank, but you are in danger of being overwhelmed with information. However, if you search for 'kidneys' you may not get many references, but by using the words 'renal' or 'urology' you will soon find relevant articles.

Key words and their synonyms help you find relevant material. When you have identified something interesting, key words are useful again: if you turn to the back of the title page in most published books and reports you will find a list of key words provided by the author for the British Library Cataloguing in Publication Data (Fig. 3.1). Compare your list with the author's to get an idea of whether the text will be useful to you.

Getting help from information technology

Information technology has revolutionized the next part of the literature search and saves a lot of time and energy. When preparing material for this edition, two hours spent at the computer terminal in the Royal College of Nursing library generated as many references as I would have gathered in two weeks manually searching indexes and abstracting journals when I was preparing the first edition. Do not be intimidated by the mention of technology; most libraries will provide the novice with an instruction sheet as to which buttons to push and when and where to type in the key words. Below are a few terms you may hear used in connection with computer-generated searches.

Data are information or facts. Therefore a **database** is a source that contains information or facts, rather like a telephone directory, but in this case, author names, titles of journals and books with a brief summary, and date of publication. The database may be a fact file, but more frequently refers to computer storage. Computerization enables searches to be made quickly because links between entries and various combinations can be identified (see the example below on stab wounds of the chest).

CD-ROM (compact disk read-only memory) is a means of storing relevant information that cannot be altered, e.g. titles, authors and summaries of research reports, journal articles or books. The disk is inserted into the computer and when you have typed in the appropriate instruction the computer will display on the terminal screen the number of references available in your chosen area.

> If you have chosen to investigate stab wounds of the chest and have typed in 'wound', you may be told there are 200–300 references or even more. This is an impossible amount of information to sort through, so you narrow or refine your field of search by entering 'stab'. (This is one area where the computer links themes.) This may still generate a large number of references, perhaps 80 or so. By being more specific still, refining the selection to 'chest', you may now be told that there are 20 references written in the last five years on stab wounds of the chest. This is a reasonable number of references to consider. By following the appropriate instructions you will be able to read the **abstract** (or summary) of each report. From this you can make a note of references that will be useful to you. Some libraries have the facility to print out the references you have chosen so that you have an accurate (and permanent) record from which to seek the article or book (Fig. 3.2).

You can see how time spent refining your ideas by discussion and identifying key words and synonyms pays dividends when you reach the computer. In some libraries the demand for computer searches is so great that time has to be booked and the length of time is limited; thus it is essential to have carried out your preparatory clarification of ideas in order to utilize your available computer time to the full.

Different organizations produce CD-ROMs; there are three or four that you are most likely to come across in nurse education libraries. However, with the rapid changes in information technology there may be others in the future.

- **MEDLINE,** produced by the US National Library of Medicine, covers over 3700 journals, includes over 8 million citations and dates back to 1966.

- **CINAHL** (Cumulative Index to Nursing and Allied Health Literature) is also produced in America, covers 700 journals and has more than 200 000 citations dating back to 1982.

```
Bookshelf                                        Catalogue Enquiry
                                                 ===============
Print requested from port OPAC14; of search 'S* 9 & 19'
================================================================
N. Author(s)  ...Title.........................Class.......Location-status ..
1 BRADEN, B J    Predictive validity of
  BERGSTROM, N   the Braden Scale for
                 pressure sore risk in
                 a nursing home population.
                 (Research) Research in
                 Nursing and Health 17(6)
                 Dec 1994 459-470
2 BURD, C and    Skin care strategies in a
  others         skilled nursing home.
                 (Research on pressure
                 sore prevention and
                 treatment) Journal of
                 Gerontological Nursing
                 20(11) Nov 1994 28-34
3 ST CLAIR, M    Tissue Viability Society.
  and others     Measuring pressure sore
                 incidence: a study.
                 (Research) Nursing
                 Standard 9, 1 Feb 1995
                 50-51
4 SHIELDS, N     Journal of Wound Care
                 Nursing. Sore concerns.
                 (Survey of pressure sores
                 in nursing homes in the
                 Eastern HSS area in
                 Northern Ireland.
                 Research) Nursing Times
                 91, 1 Feb 1995 68, 70, 72
5 HALFENS, R J G Knowledge, beliefs and
                 use of nursing methods in
  EGGINK, M      preventing pressure sores
                 in Dutch hospitals.
                 (Research) International
                 Journal of Nursing
                 Studies 32(1) Feb 1995
                 16-26
6 BONNEFOY, M    Implication of cytokines
  and others     in the aggravation of
                 malnutrition and
                 hypercatabolism in
                 elderly patients with
                 severe pressure sores.
                 (Research) Age and Ageing
                 24(1) Jan 1995 37-42
```

Figure 3.2   Example of printout from literature search on pressure sores.

- **RCN Nurse ROM** was produced by the Royal College of Nursing. The fifth and final issues were released in March 1997.

- **British Nursing Index (BNI)** started in January 1997 and consolidates *Nursing Bibliography*, RCN Nurse ROM and NMI (Nursing and Midwifery Index). The database includes over 220 health-related journals, many from the UK. It is anticipated that 9000 references will be added each year. The BNI is produced in three formats: on the Internet, by subscription; CD-ROM available quarterly; and in printed form, with 12 issues a year and an annual cumulation.

For those of you with access to the ***Internet/Web site*** you will find many pages very useful, such as the ENB (English National Board) Home Page. The ENB Home Page contains circulars, research papers, information leaflets and many other aspects relevant to nursing. Other examples include the RCN Home Page and home pages for several journals and universities, even departments within universities. Additionally, the Internet can provide access to research and discussions of research, often from all over the world, especially the USA.

Research has been carried out into the usefulness of MEDLINE and CINAHL in nursing literature searches. Brazier and Begley (1996) concluded that there was no difference in the two databases overall but the references in MEDLINE were significantly more accessible in all aspects of nursing, except the organization of nursing.

Further help

If you need to search the literature for information prior to the 1980s, then you will need to do a manual search using various indexes or specialized *abstracting journals*. Again, the key words are helpful when you search abstracting journals. An abstracting journal is a publication that summarizes published material in a particular subject area. The most useful for you is likely to be *Nursing Research Abstracts*, which was published by the Department of Health and Social Security four times a year. Many nursing libraries will still have copies, although the last issue was vol. 16 no. 4 in 1994. Publication ceased as it was felt that CD-ROMs had made the abstracts obsolete. Prior to the release of RCN Nurse ROM, the information was contained in the *Nursing Bibliography*, which was published by the Royal College of Nursing every two months and listed published nursing texts. Not all the titles listed were research publications, so be careful if you are seeking research findings.

You may have a friendly librarian who will do the literature search for you. If you are a member of the Royal College of Nursing the College Library will carry out a search for you if you cannot get to the library in person, although there may be a time delay depending on demand. If you are a student at university there are likely to be facilities available to you on the campus. However, Moorbath (1995) reports a worrying decline in access and availability of libraries to nurses. He concludes his study by saying that the number of nursing library sites has fallen over the last few years and in 20% of cases surveyed the distance between college sites and libraries is over 10 miles. However, in the remaining 80% there has been an improvement in facilities with access to new technologies. Moorbath states that the fewer remaining libraries have the opportunity to offer more professional services that small, unstaffed or partly staffed libraries cannot. If you have to travel, make sure you are well organized and clear about what you wish to find out. Finally, ensure that your briefing is as precise as possible. Make it clear how far back you wish the search to go: just the last 5 years or the last 40? Make sure you stipulate which languages you are fluent in: I failed to do this in my ward sister–learning search and ended up with an article in Japanese and two in German. Fortunately a student nurse was able to translate the Japanese article and a relative translated the German articles.

Starting to read

Once you have four or five references, I suggest you start reading. Always read the most recent article or book first as there will be useful references taking you back through the literature to yet more references. Once your reading is underway you will soon find that the real problem is not difficulty in getting references but the potential for being overwhelmed by a pile of paper. Again your key words help you keep to your original aim see Chapter 4 and stop you from being side-tracked. The next chapter considers how you can stay up to date with all the reading and information. All the new references in this second edition have been taken from journals and material that were available in my local nurse library. I have selected examples that are in nursing journals commonly held in nurse libraries so that you should be able to access them easily, although they do not necessarily represent the most in-depth or detailed study on the topic.

4

Making records

Key words:
- References
- Bibliographic software

Whether you are reading in the comfort of your own home or in a library, it is wise to follow these steps before you go any further.

First, record details of what you are reading. However time-consuming or irritating this may seem, take care to record accurately and in detail. This might be a chore now but in a few weeks or months, when you come to write an essay or share your information with another, you will be glad you spent the time!

Where to record these details

Your records may be handwritten or stored in a computer. First I discuss using index cards and then look at how a hand-held or laptop computer can make life easier.

The written version

I prefer to use lined index cards 20 × 12 cm (though various sizes are available from most stationers). These should be stored somewhere safe, and in alphabetical order for easy retrieval. An old shoe box might be a suitable storage box or you can buy file boxes or drawers for your cards if you prefer. Index cards are small enough to carry around but large enough to contain essential information. Record each article or report on a separate card. Even record articles and reports you have looked at and decided are not relevant to your work now – they may be later! Or they may be useful to someone else.

Write your key words on one of the cards so that you have a written record of them to remind you of your objective.

Information technology

Generating, storing and using recorded information is made easier if you have a hand-held or laptop computer: you can enter data directly while reading. This can then be transferred to your home computer, where you can build up a bank of **references** and information that is quickly accessible and easily manipulated into various formats for essay and project writing. Commercial software packages such as Procite, Reference Manager and Endnote are available and compatible with various types of computers. This **bibliographic software** for personal collections of references has made the task of filing and searching for relevant references very easy. Most systems enable you to identify the references you require from those you have recorded and will format them in the style required by your college or publisher. I have cited just three software packages that are available; however, information technology is a volatile market, which means rapid changes in **software** and **hardware** (the computer itself). Finally, an important point: remember to make a back-up copy in case of computer failure or power cuts, which can cause havoc with some systems.

What information should be recorded

1. Author's surname and initials. These will be found on the title page (Fig. 4.1 (A)). If a book has chapters by different authors, the author's name will be given after the chapter title.

2. Editor's name and initials (if it is a book of chapters from different contributors) will be found on the title page.

3. Year published. This occurs on the bibliographic page, which is usually the reverse of the title page (Fig. 4.2 (B)). Note that it is the date of publication *not* the date of the last reprint (i.e. in Fig. 4.2, (B) not (C)).

4. Title of book and subtitles (Fig. 4.1 (D)).

5. Edition, if not the first (Fig. 4.1 (E)).

6. Number of pages, if only part of a book is used.

7. Place of publication and publisher (Figs 4.1 (F) and 4.2 (G)).

Figure 4.3 shows an example of a completed record card.

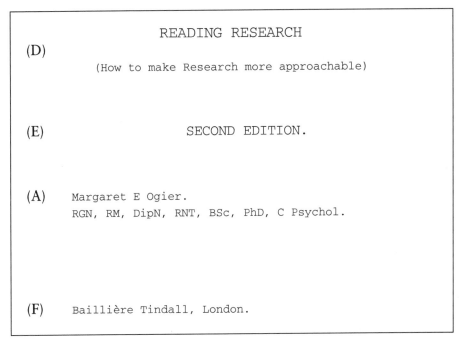

Figure 4.1   Sample title page.

The procedure is a little more complicated for articles in journals:

1. Author's surname and initials.
2. Year of publication.
3. Title of article and subtitles.
4. Journal title.
5. Volume and part numbers.
6. The inclusive page numbers of the article.
7. Date of publication.

Figure 4.4 shows an example of a completed record card for a journal article.

A tip that you may find useful, whether you are using manual or computer recording, is to note where you obtained the reference, journal article or book. I use the right-hand corner of the index card for this (see Figs 4.3 and 4.4). If it is my own copy I use an asterisk, if I borrowed it from a friend or colleague I put

(G) Scutari Press

Viking House, 17–19 Peterborough Road,
Harrow, Middlesex HA1 2AX, England

A division of Scutari Projects, the publishing company of
the Royal College of Nursing

(B) © Scutari Press 1989

All rights reserved. No part of this publication may be reproduced, stored in a retrieval system or transmitted, in any form or by any means, electronic, mechanical, photocopying or otherwise, without the prior permission of Scutari Press, Viking House, 17–19 Peterborough Road, Harrow, Middlesex HA1 2AX, England.

(C) First published 1989
Reprinted 1989, 1990, 1991, 1992

British Library Cataloguing in Publication Data

Ogier, Margaret E
Reading research
1. Medicine. Nursing
I. Title
610.73

ISBN 1–871364–02–7

Typeset by Photo·graphics, Honiton, Devon
Printed in Great Britain by Queensbury Press Ltd., London

Figure 4.2 Sample bibliographic detail page.

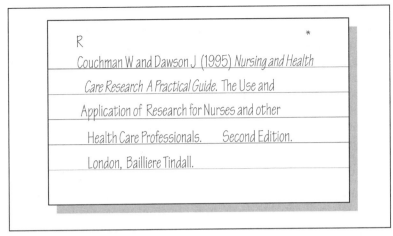

Figure 4.3   *Completed record card for a book reference.*

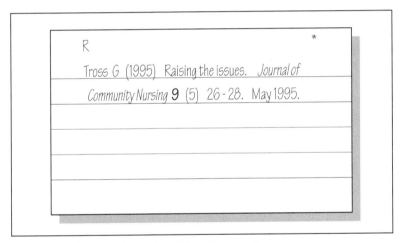

Figure 4.4   *Completed record card for a journal reference.*

their name; if I obtained it from a library, I put the library's name. If it is a library copy, besides putting the name or initials of the library you borrowed it from (e.g. Royal College of Nursing, RCN), you can also put the class and accession numbers. This may seem like a lot of extra work before you even start the task of reading, but in two or three months' time when you refer to your cards and want more details on a particular aspect you can retrieve the original report without too much difficulty.

The final piece of information to be recorded on the card must wait until you have read the article or report. You can then use the top left-hand corner to indicate the subject matter of the article, e.g. 'man' to indicate 'management', 'n man' to indicate 'nursing management', etc. You can use any categories that are relevant to you. Use one of your cards to record your abbreviations, otherwise when you return to your cards after a few months you may not remember whether 'cc' stands for 'catheter care' or 'coronary care'. Similar information can be stored on computer, depending on what software you are using.

All this takes time, but in the long term it will allow you to easily retrieve articles if you want to refresh your memory on some aspect or find information for an essay or project. In this respect, information technology will help you greatly.

The way you are required to reference your work will usually be stipulated by your course director or publishers. There are two frequently used referencing systems. The first is called the Harvard system, which is used in this book: the author's name and date appear in the text, with the full references in alphabetical order at the end of the chapter or book. The other is called the Vancouver system: a number is placed in the text where a reference occurs, with the references listed in numerical order at the end of the chapter or book.

With all this work completed you can now start to read and appraise your chosen report. Chapters 5–9 consider sections of the report as you are likely to encounter them.

5
Making sense of reports

Key words:
- Abstract
- Report layout

It is far easier to read something if you have some idea of what it is about. Authors of research reports are aware of this and want to attract the reader, so they usually preface the report with an **abstract** (a summary of why the study was done and the main results). If you are reading a journal article, the abstract usually takes the form of a paragraph at the start of the article. Such a paragraph may be set in a different typeface to attract your attention (Fig. 5.1). In theses and research reports, the first page is usually devoted to the abstract.

Read the abstract through several times to get an idea of what you are about to read. If you are using your own copy, you may like to underline or highlight key words. If you are using a borrowed copy, write the key words on your index card or enter them into your computerized record.

If you are still not sure what the report is about, turn to the end and read the conclusion or summary several times, again identifying key words.

Now you have some idea about the report, but do *not* think that this is enough and you can skip the tedious bit in the middle! If you do, you may find that you have come to the wrong conclusions. For the next part bring your knowledge and common sense into play and use the pointers provided in this book to help you read critically. You need to use your own experience and knowledge to formulate questions about what you are reading.

Journal of Psychiatric and Mental Health Nursing, 1996, **3,** 61-66

Reasons for non-attendance at a day hospital for people with enduring mental illness: the clients' perspective

1. M. McGONAGLE RMN, DIPN (CPN)[1]; J. GENTLE RMN, RGN, RCNT, BSC (HONS)[2]

1 *Audery House, Southern Derbyshire Mental Trust*
2 *University of Nottingham, Faculty of Medicine and Health Science, School of Nursing and Midwifery, Derby, UK*

Correspondence:
Mrs Jan Gentle
University of Nottingham and
Midwifery
Melbourne House
96 Osmaston Road
Derby DE1 2RD
UK

McGONAGLE I. M. & GENTLE J. (1996) *Journal of Psychiatric and Mental Health Nursing* **3,** 61-66.
Reasons for non-attendance at a day hospital for people with enduring mental health nursing: the clients' perspective

This paper describes a research project which aimed to discover the reasons clients give for failing to attend a mental health day hospital. There was concern that this service provision, for people with enduring mental illness, had a high level of non-attendance and therfore might not be meeting the needs of people for whom it is targeted. Over a period of 6 months 36 people failed to attend, despite assessment and apparent agreement to attend. Of the 36, 14 agreed to talk about their reasons for not attending. An open interview format was used which enabled the clients to talk in depth about their experiences, which they felt led to the decision to stop attending. Content analysis of the interview data resulted in the identification of common themes. Main findings suggest a lack of partnership in decisions on choice of therapy, particulaly the emphasis on groupwork, which resulted 86% found unhelpful. Other main factors for non-attendance were a lack of an individual approach to care, not being listened to, and a lack of warmth form the staff. Recommendations for future pratice are given, with particular attention to the need to develop a partnership with clients aimed at meeting individual needs.

Abstract

Note use of Keywords

Keywords: day service, non-attendance, partnership, qulitative, research, user voice

Accepted for publication: 23 August 1995

Background

Since national plans to scale down mental health inpatient facilities were announced some years ago attention has focused on the development of community provision, along with the concern that this should be used as effectively and efficiently as possible. This study is concerned with the level of non-attendance at a day hospital for people with enduring mental illness, and users' reasons for non-attendance are explored.

Literature is available on the nature of mental health day hospital provision and there is a genral agreement that the focus should be on people with enduring severe mental illness. It has also been identified that, for this client group, behavioural

approaches and social activites are found to be more benefical than dynamic therapeutic interventions, (Falloon & Talbot 1982, Milne 1984, Thornicroft & Bebbington 1989, Holloway 1991).

There appears to be little written on the reasons for high non-attendance rates. However, Carter (1981), in a national study services, found an average underattendance level of 40%. Strachaan and Stuckey's (1989) survey on patient's early experiences of the day hospital treatment suggests possible reasons for non-engagement at a day hospital in Edinburgh (where the level of non-attendance was 33% over a 2-year period). These included patients seeing themselves as too well to need such treatment; a lack of drive and volition experienced by individuals with schizophrenia; anxiety about meeting new people; and fear of what

Figure 5.1   Abstract. (From McGonagle, M. and Gentle, J. (1996) Journal of Psychiatric and Mental Health Nursing **3,** *61–66. With permission of Blackwell Science.)*

Pathways and stepping stones through a research report

There is a common format to research reports. The first two parts (which we have already mentioned) are the *title*, followed by an *abstract*. The other sections or parts of a report are listed here to give you an overall picture; however, each part is the subject of a separate chapter.

- *Introduction.* This gives the background to the study and tells you why the particular piece of research was undertaken. A brief résumé of previous and related work will also be given, either in the introduction or possibly under a separate heading, *Literature Review*, which will be helpful to you with your own literature search as the background literature is discussed. see Chapter 6

- *Method or Methodology.* This is an account of how the study was carried out. see Chapter 7

- *Results.* This is usually a short factual section in which the findings of the study are depicted, often with graphs and tables. see Chapter 8

- *Discussion.* In this section the author discusses the findings of the study in the light of previous work, described in the literature review, and other relevant issues. see Chapter 9

- *Conclusion.* The author summarizes the study, drawing the threads together and perhaps indicating the strengths, weaknesses and implications for use of the study. see Chapter 9

- *References.* All studies mentioned in the text should be listed in detail. You should be able to access any of these relatively easily if the references have been presented correctly.

- *Appendices* contain material of interest relevant to the study itself, but not included in the body of the report (e.g. the questionnaire or interview schedule used during the research).

You now have an overview of the **layout** or order of presentation of a research report. Depending on whether you are reading an article in a journal or an original thesis, you will find that the parts vary in the amount of detail covered (ranging from a few lines to several chapters) but the basic format will be the same. However, you should be aware of the enormous difference in depth and detail between a thesis and a 2000-word report written for publication in a journal. If the article is based on a thesis, the full document will be cited in the references or acknowledged in a note at the beginning of the article.

The headings in a report are an important guide to answering an essential question: Is this an account of a research study or

---

RESEARCH REPORT SUMMARY

Title of study:

Authors:

Date of study: Date of publication:

Aim of study:

Research questions and/or hypotheses:

Sample and sample size:

Method of study and research tools used:

Results:

Conclusions of the study:

Figure 5.2   Research report summary form.

someone's views and opinions? There are many interesting, well-informed journal articles and books written by well-known authors, but however good they may be they are not necessarily research reports. If you have been asked to write a critique of a piece of research, or if you are using evidence to justify a nursing decision or action, you need to know if it is an actual research report or merely a knowledgeable account of facts and opinions. Any material that fits clearly into the above headings is likely to be a piece of research. This distinction is important as nursing moves forwards to become an evidence-based profession. You will not be able to make any firm judgement about the quality of the research, the appropriateness of the techniques used, or the veracity of the writer's conclusions. These are skills you will need to develop and I hope that by the time you have read the research, with this book as a guide, you will be more informed and critical in your reading.

To help clarify your thoughts prepare an A4 summary sheet with the headings shown in Fig. 5.2. You may feel that this is duplicating your index card. However, when you start reading research reports you may have difficulty picking out the salient points so that they fit on to the index card. You can summarize the points on the A4 sheet and transpose them to the index card at the end of the exercise.

Developing a questioning attitude to what you read

Now that you have read the abstract and the conclusions you should have an idea of what the study is about. Earlier I warned you to be careful not to fall into the trap of thinking that this will be enough.

Completing the first part of the summary sheet with the title, author and date of publication should be easy enough. What may not be apparent immediately, however, is the date when the study was *actually* carried out (as opposed to the publication date of the report). The date of the study may only become apparent as you read the introduction. On occasions, the only way I have discovered when the work was done was from material in the appendices, such as dated letters or questionnaires. You may wonder why it is important to be concerned about when exactly the research was done. This is because there is always a gap between writing and publishing, often as long as

18 months to two years. There may have been an even longer gap between completion of the research and the writing of the report or article! Some areas of nursing are changing quickly, such as the facilities for day surgery or non-invasive investigations, so the information in the report may be out of date before it is published or it may have been superseded by more up-to-

---

RESEARCH REPORT SUMMARY

Title of study: Reasons for non-attendance at a day hospital for people with enduring mental illness: the clients' perspective.

Authors: McGonagle I M and Gentle J.

Date of study: 31st July 95.   Date of publication: 1996

Aim of study: was to discover the reasons why clients decided to stop attending a mental health day hospital for people with enduring mental illness.

Research questions and/or hypotheses: not given, inferred in the aim.

Sample and sample size: Non attenders at day hospital 36, 18m, 18f. Only 14 agreed to be interviewed.

Method of study and research tools used: Unstructured interviews, recorded, carried out by a nurse but not one involved in day hospital. Content analysis of interview by the two researchers.
    Groupwork unhelpful 86%.
    Lack of individual approach 57%.
    Staff did not listen 42%.
    Feeling forgotten 36%.
    Lack of warmth (emotional) 36%.
    Lack of support 29%.

Discussion: Lack of choice in therapeutic approaches to group work; feel care did not take note of individual needs and that those needs were not listened to.

Conclusions: Six recommendations formulated.

Figure 5.3   Sample of completed research report summary form.

date knowledge. This does *not* mean that the report should not be read. There is still a possibility that it will provide valuable insights. However, it does mean that if you are considering implementing the findings or changing your practice as a result of your reading, you must be aware of how current the research actually is.

An example of a completed summary sheet for the journal article used in Fig. 5.1 is shown in Fig. 5.3.

Each of the following chapters addresses a section of the research report. You should always be prepared to ask questions about what you are reading. Some questions are given in each chapter to help get you started.

Special terms, used in research reports in a more precise manner than in general speech, are set in bold type and are defined in the Glossary. Not all the terms may be found in any one report and not all possible terms are covered in this book. However, more detailed texts are suggested in the Further reading at the end of this book.

6

The introduction and literature review

Key words:
- Literature review
- Hypothesis
- Null hypothesis

The introduction usually includes a statement of why the research was done. The **literature review** gives an overview of previous research or writings on the topic. In a research report or thesis this will form a separate chapter/section but in a journal article it may be covered in the first few paragraphs.

As mentioned in the previous chapter there are essential questions a reader needs to ask in order to develop skills of critical appraisal.

- What was the aim of the study? Fill this in on your A4 summary sheet. You will need to refer to the aim on several occasions while you are reading to remind yourself what the researcher was trying to study. For instance, when you get to the results section, do the results agree with the aim? And you will need to check the aim against the conclusions. You might even want to refer to the aim while reading the methodology and consider whether you would have used the same processes to find answers to the stipulated purpose of the study.

The literature review usually presents studies and reports that have informed the researcher and provides the background or foundation upon which the present study is based. The literature review leads into either the research questions or hypotheses.

see
Chapter 1

■ What was the research question being asked? At the beginning of this book, we examined the aim of my research study, which was about the influence of ward sisters on student nurses. After discussion, the research question was developed into a form for which answers could be sought. My study was a descriptive study to find out about ward sister–student nurse interactions. As the study progressed and answers began to form in response to the research questions, so it became possible to formulate hypotheses.

Hypothesis

A **hypothesis** (plural, hypotheses) is a statement based on knowledge or information that has yet to be proved or disproved. In a seminal piece of nursing research, Boore (1978) gives two experimental hypotheses:

1. 'The preoperative giving of information about postoperative treatment and care, and teaching exercises to be performed postoperatively, will minimise the rise in biochemical indicators of stress.'

2. 'A relationship will be demonstrated between the measurements of biochemical indicators of stress and some other indicators of patient welfare.'

Null hypothesis

A **null hypothesis** states that there will be *no significant difference* between the control and the experimental groups. Using an experimental research design, the researcher sets out to gather data that will support or disprove this hypothesis. For example, Kerr *et al.* (1996) used an experimental design to study whether providing parents with advice in the postnatal period would reduce sleep problems in infants. Their null hypothesis was that 'there was no statistically significant difference in the sleeping behaviour of the control group and the intervention group'. The null hypothesis was rejected. Therefore, advice in the postnatal period does appear to be beneficial in preventing sleep problems in infants.

Be careful when you are reading your research report as it is easy to come to the wrong conclusion. If the experimental hypothesis is supported, the meaning will be exactly opposite to what it would be if the null hypothesis was supported. In both the Boore (1978) and Kerr *et al.* (1996) studies the hypotheses were supported, which means that preoperative information *does* minimize the biochemical indicators of stress and postnatal advice *does* reduce sleep problems in infants. A study by Sleep (1988), investigating whether salt in the bath affected the healing of episiotomies, found that 90% of mothers found no difference whether they used salt or not. In Sleep's study the null hypothesis was supported, showing that salt in bath water does *not* significantly affect wound healing. So be careful with your reading and check which hypothesis has been supported.

■ In the study you are reading has the researcher posed a hypothesis? Is the hypothesis relevant to the question being asked or to the aim of the study?

Not all research studies have hypotheses. My study, using a grounded theory approach, started with the aim of describing what sisters were doing to improve or impede learning in the clinical area. Only as the study advanced and differences between medical and surgical ward sisters became apparent did I formulate a hypothesis. Grahn and Danielson (1996), evaluating an education and support programme for cancer patients, also used a grounded theory approach to their descriptive study as they felt it was a research design sensitive to the topic and where testing hypotheses would be inappropriate. The next chapter considers different ways of carrying out research in order to meet the aims of the study, in other words the method or methodology.

7
The method or methodology

Both *method* and *methodology* relate to the way in which the researcher tried to fulfil the aim of the study you have just identified in the report you are reading. Methodology includes such aspects as **research design** used, **sample** size and selection, **research tools** used and ways of collecting and analysing data. You might also at this point think about the **ethical** considerations and implications of the research you are studying (see for example de Raeve 1996).

There are various ways of classifying research but perhaps the most helpful approach is to consider the three main types of research that you are likely to encounter:

- descriptive research
- experimental research
- action research.

You will also encounter research that is quantitative or

qualitative or a mixture of both. There is no shortage of articles and discussion on the pros and cons of each type of research.

G ▶ **Quantitative research** is more concerned with collecting and analysing data that focus on numbers and frequencies rather than on meaning or experience. Hence it is often referred to as 'number crunching'! This type of research is mainly associated with experimental designs such as those used by Kerr *et al.* (1996).

G ▶ **Qualitative research** is mainly descriptive and involves the collection and analysis of data concerned with meanings, attitudes and beliefs rather than data that results in numerical counts from which statistical inferences can be drawn. For example, see the studies by Waterman *et al.* (1996), who evaluated the introduction of case management on a newly created rehabilitation floor at an elderly care hospital, or Spouse (1990), who sought ways of improving the quality of the learning environment for student nurses in clinical areas. Qualitative research tends to generate a lot of evidence that requires analysis and this can be problematical: how do you analyse people's opinions? Russell and Gregory (1993) have produced some answers to this question that include both manual and information technology methods, but that discussion is beyond the scope of this book.

Some researchers use both quantitative and qualitative methods, e.g. the study by Barrett *et al.* (1996) used a descriptive design that included both quantitative and qualitative data while evaluating a baccalaureate nursing programme.

One method is not better than another; what is important is that the method of research most appropriate to the aim of the study is chosen. This is where you use your knowledge and nursing experience to question whether the method chosen seems to be the sensible choice. Russell and Gregory (1993) comment that qualitative research has 'come of age' and it is now accepted that qualitative research can be an end in itself not just the prelude to a 'proper' quantitative study.

■ Is the report you are reading quantitative, qualitative or a mixture of both?

Descriptive research

The researcher tries to describe accurately (to paint a picture in words and figures) the findings derived from careful, systematic collection and recording of information or data. Many nursing studies are descriptive. Nursing research is still 'young' and there are many aspects of nursing that need to be studied and described. The different ways data are gathered are numerous and often referred to as research tools; these include **question-naires, interviews** and **observations**. The different types of tool, together with their advantages and disadvantages, are discussed in more detail later in the chapter. First, some different descriptive studies are explained briefly in order to show how these techniques can be used to inform nurses.

> Atkinson and Sklaroff (1987) studied the care provided for 75 physically disabled patients admitted to acute general hospital wards. They were also interested to see how hospitalization had affected their well-being on return home. The study shows that the layout of the wards, nursing routines and inadequate nurse–patient communication resulted in the disabled patients being more dependent than they need have been.
>
> Barrett et al. (1996) wanted to find out if graduates from a nursing programme felt they had achieved their end-of-course objectives and whether those objectives met the employer's needs. By analysing the responses of the students and employers they were able to conclude the course was satisfactory.
>
> Coates (1985) used a descriptive **cross-sectional study** to examine the nutritional status of patients in wards that were organized differently, rather than the same ward over months or years. Hicks et al. (1996) used semi-structured interviews to gather information about attitudes to research from six members of four primary health teams, again obtaining a cross-section of opinions.
>
> Rather than using a cross-sectional design, some researchers use **longitudinal studies** that examine the same group of people over time. Kirkevold et al. (1996) used a short time-span (8 weeks) when they studied the recovery of heart surgery patients, whereas Jerrett and Costello (1996) spent two years gathering data from parents of asthmatic children and describing how they did or did not gain control of the situation.

Experimental research

This type of research is useful for establishing a relationship between cause and effect. In Chapter 6, we looked at two studies that used experimental design when we considered hypotheses: both Boore (1978) and Kerr *et al.* (1996) used an experimental design to see whether information-giving would result in a reduced problem, i.e. postoperative stress and sleep problems in infants, respectively.

It is usual when embarking on an experimental research project to divide the group of people or things, **subjects**, into subgroups that are as similar as possible. One subgroup, the **experimental group**, experiences the factor under considera-tion. The second subgroup, the **control group**, does *not* experience the particular factor. If the two groups do not dif-fer in any other way, any change that occurs in the experi-mental group but *not* in the control group would appear to be due to the introduced factor. This factor may be referred to as a **variable**.

The **independent variable** is the experimental factor that is deliberately manipulated. In Boore (1978) and Kerr *et al.* (1996), the independent variable was the level of information given to the experimental group but not to the control group.

The **dependent variable** is the aspect being studied to see if the experimental factor has any effect. In Boore (1978) the dependent variable was postoperative stress while in Kerr *et al.* (1996) it was the sleep problems of infants.

When you are reading reports of experimental research it is important to remember what the variables are. One way of doing this is to write each one out on a card, labelling them independent or dependent, and then to use the card as a book-mark as you read through the report. When presenting results or discussing their findings many authors refer to dependent or independent variables (but not what they were), so you are fre-quently having to refer back to make sure you are not getting confused. Writing the variables on a card saves time and reduces your frustration levels! The study of Kerr *et al.* (1996) is examined briefly below.

An example of an experimental study is Kerr et al. (1996). One of the commonest problems in the preschool child that causes parents to seek advice from health professionals is the sleepless child. Disturbed sleep puts the parents under stress and in some cases places the child at risk of abuse. Kerr et al. wished to find out if health education could reduce the incidence of sleep problems. Participants were randomly allocated to either the control group or the intervention, experimental, group of 90 and 100 subjects; hence the term **randomized controlled trial**. The intervention group were given specific information on sleep patterns and settling methods when babies were three months old. The sleeping behaviour of both groups was compared six months later when the babies were nine months old. The intervention group were sleeping better with less problems.

■ What are the variables being considered in Kerr et al.'s study? (See end of this chapter, on page 52, for the answer.)

Action research

In action research, researchers pay attention to a particular problem or change they wish to bring about in one specific situation. In carrying out most research, researchers try *not* to alter the situation, other than the independent variable. However, once subjects are informed of a research study the situation alters in subtle ways; with action research, the researcher sets out to alter the situation! Researchers observe in a systematic manner the way the problem is solved or change is implemented. A useful article by Waterman (1995) considers the differences between, and similarities of, 'traditional' and action research. A few examples of action research studies may help to clarify this research design or method.

Fretwell (1982) carried out a descriptive study in which she identified wards that were good teaching wards for student nurses and those that were less good. She followed this up with an action research study in which she developed a programme, based in the wards, to help sisters who had problems with creating a learning environment in the clinical area. In this way she introduced change, watched and documented what happened, and reported it in *Freedom to Change* (Fretwell, 1985).

Since Fretwell's pioneering work with action research in nursing during the 1980s, other nurse researchers have used this method with success in a variety of nursing areas. West (1992) used an action research framework to change nursing staff's management of pressure sores into a research-based approach, which focused on the nutrition of the elderly. East and Robinson (1994) considered how best to bring about change, especially at ward level, and chose an action research design. The study identified that general managers and professionals have different agendas for change but there was common ground. Newton (1995) reviewed the use of action research in nursing and used action research to look at the effects of the care planning element of the computerized integrated Hospital Information System (HIS) on ward nurses in a district general hospital.

It can be seen from these references that the use of action research is increasing and is particularly useful in areas related to change. Waterman (1995) provides a starting point for those interested in such a debate and draws on various schema and criteria from which to judge the functionality and effectiveness of action research. The journal *Nurse Researcher*, vol. 2, no. 3, March 1995 is devoted to a discussion of this topic and from which you can identify further references if you are particularly interested in this method of research.

Ethnography and phenomenology

As nursing moves closer to becoming a research-based profession and to use evidence-based practice, so the types of design used in nursing research increase. For instance, you may come across reports such as Jan Savage's *Nursing Intimacy: an Ethnographic Approach to Nurse–Patient Interaction* (Savage,

1995). This study explores what nurses understand by the notion of 'closeness' and to assess the support they might need where 'close' relationships with patients are encouraged. So how did she carry out the study and what does 'Ethnography' mean? There are various definitions of **ethnography**; fortunately Ballie (1995) has provided a comprehensive review of the origins and development of ethnography as a research approach in nursing. In essence, ethnography is a flexible method in which the researcher participates in people's lives, collecting data in order to provide an explanation for the chosen topic. Ethnography focuses on understanding the perspectives of the people being studied and observes them in everyday life rather than in artificial or experimental conditions. This is basically a descriptive methodology, while **phenomenology** is an interpretative methodology that examines subject's perceptions of their own experiences. The researcher attempts to present these perceptions with clarity and to interpret their structure and meaning. Phenomenology is a qualitative approach to research and for some is still controversial. However, as it records the subject's perceptions, this could be a valuable way of studying patients, their needs and nursing care. If you want to know more, Hallett (1995) is a most useful article. In the future there will be yet more research designs introduced for you to come to terms with, but for the moment we have looked at the main current designs that you will encounter in your reading.

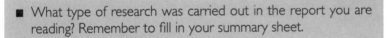

■ What type of research was carried out in the report you are reading? Remember to fill in your summary sheet.

Sample and sample size

After defining the research questions and choosing an appropriate type of research method, the author will need to decide on a *sample* and on the *size of the sample*. Both of these will be influenced by the research questions and the research design chosen. A sample is a selection of people from the possible **population**, e.g. eight ward sisters from a total of 24 sisters working in hospital A.

The systematic selection of a sample to ensure that all

possible members of the population stand an equal chance of being selected is known as a **random sampling**. For example, if all 24 sisters were willing to take part in the study but time and money meant that only eight could take part, then to ensure each had a chance of being chosen all their names would be written on pieces of paper and put into a hat and eight pieces of paper drawn out. Thus each sister would have an equal chance of being selected.

■ What was the sample size in the report you are reading? Remember to fill in your summary sheet.
■ How does the sample size relate to the possible population?

An example showing the importance of sample size is shown below.

Six patients with anxiety neurosis were observed for half a day when there were 40 similar patients attending the same day clinic.

■ What was the significance of the length of time for which they were observed?
■ Was it long enough?
■ Was there any special significance to the date chosen?
■ Was there a marked deviation from the usual routine that day?

If the aim of the study was to observe whether variation in routine caused an increase in a particular behaviour in specific patients, then the number and date chosen might be appropriate. However, if the aim of the study was to describe typical daily activities of patients with anxiety neurosis on a typical day, then the sample size and timing could be questioned.

Now you can see why it is important for you to establish the aim of the study, as it has implications for the methods used, sample size, method of data collection, etc. Some examples of the sample size used in different studies are shown below.

Ragneskog *et al.* (1996) used video observation of five demented patients to assess the effect of music on their behaviour. Just five patients provided a lot of qualitative data. Using data that had been collected for an antenatal care project, Clement *et al.* (1996) analysed 1882 maternity records, while Runciman *et al.* (1996) looked at 414 patients over 75 years of age who attended an accident and emergency department and considered the effects of health visitor intervention.

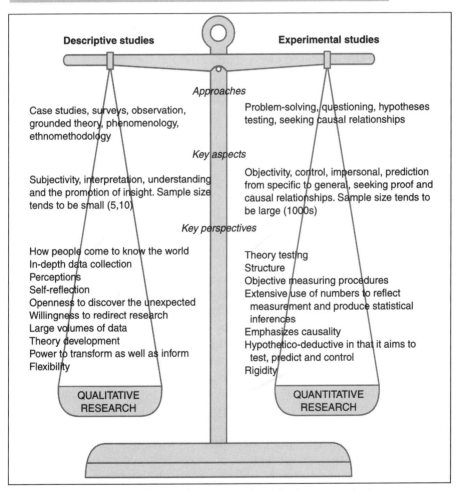

Descriptive studies   **Experimental studies**

Approaches

Case studies, surveys, observation, grounded theory, phenomenology, ethnomethodology

Problem-solving, questioning, hypotheses testing, seeking causal relationships

Key aspects

Subjectivity, interpretation, understanding and the promotion of insight. Sample size tends to be small (5,10)

Objectivity, control, impersonal, prediction from specific to general, seeking proof and causal relationships. Sample size tends to be large (1000s)

Key perspectives

How people come to know the world
In-depth data collection
Perceptions
Self-reflection
Openness to discover the unexpected
Willingness to redirect research
Large volumes of data
Theory development
Power to transform as well as inform
Flexibility

Theory testing
Structure
Objective measuring procedures
Extensive use of numbers to reflect measurement and produce statistical inferences
Emphasizes causality
Hypothetico-deductive in that it aims to test, predict and control
Rigidity

QUALITATIVE RESEARCH

QUANTITATIVE RESEARCH

Figure 7.1   The weighting of various factors towards qualitative or quantitative research. This is depicted as a set of pan scales, since there is no rigid divide between the two approaches, rather a changing balance between the varying philosophies of research and the methods employed.

Volume 3, no. 4 of *Nurse Researcher* (June 1996) is devoted to sampling. If you feel in doubt about the size of the sample in the report you are reading then you can find more detailed accounts of many aspects of sampling in this special issue, although some of the articles are complex.

Figure 7.1 depicts the methodological issues related to quantitative and qualitative research.

Pilot study

Usually a preliminary study or **pilot study** will be carried out to test the proposed method and research tools for the main study. Sometimes this pilot study will be described in the Methodology section, or it can provide enough material for a journal article, e.g. Stonehouse and Butcher (1996) and Dubyna and Quinn (1996).

The pilot study might identify problems in the choice of method or in the research tools, necessitating a change of plans. You are likely to come across instances in full research reports but not in journal articles. This is a good reason to make sure you read the whole report, not just the summary and the conclusions!

Research tools

These include questionnaires, audio and video recordings, interview schedules or observations. Observations can be behavioural or physiological, such as weight or skinfold thickness, participant or non-participant.

Participant observation is when the researcher is also part of what is being observed, e.g. when a staff nurse in a surgical ward observes the number of times student nurses spontaneously initiate conversation with patients aged over 70 years.

Non-participant observation is when the researcher is not part of the situation being observed.

All these research tools are ways of collecting data or information.

- How was data collected in the study you are reading? Remember to record it on your summary sheet.
- With regard to the stated aim of the study you are reading and your nursing knowledge and common sense, was the most appropriate method used?
- If you do not think the method the most appropriate, why was it used? What would have been better?
- If you had used the same research tools as the author of the report would you have used them in the same way?

There are two important points that you should keep in mind when questioning the use of any research tool: it must have reliability and validity.

Reliability assesses the degree to which the tool is measuring something, but good reliability does not mean that the tool is measuring what it is supposed to measure! **Validity** is concerned with whether the tool measures what it is supposed to measure. There are various ways of testing that research tools are reliable and valid. If you are reading a journal article there may only be a passing mention that reliability and validity were verified, whereas research reports and theses should describe how the tools used were tested for reliability and validity.

Reliability is typically assessed by looking at the match (*correlation*) between two sets of scores when the same tool is used with the same group of people on two occasions. If the scores correlate, this is known as **temporal stability** (or test–retest reliability). Sometimes two forms of the same tool yield similar scores; this is referred to as *alternate form reliability*. Other researchers test for **internal consistency** of the research tool they plan to use by looking at how separate parts within the tool correlate; this is done by looking at the scores of the individual parts compared with the overall scores. In nursing there are times when nurses have to use their judgement about patients' behaviour or condition. The reliability of such assessments is tested by using two assessors and comparing their scores using a test of correlation, which provides an index of **interscorer/interjudge reliability**.

Validity is assessed by correlating the score with some external criterion to obtain a *validity coefficient*. For example, if a test was designed to assess student nurses' ability to complete a course successfully, these scores would be correlated with their course marks and a match or correlation sought. This kind of validity is called **criterion (empirical) validity. Construct validity** refers to a tool that has been designed to measure some concept which forms part of a theory and that has been found to be valid in the process of theory testing. To be satisfied of a tool's construct validity, several different ways of testing the tool and the theory are carried out.

So, does the research tool used in the study actually measure what it is supposed to do (validity) in a consistent manner (reliability)? If you are reading a journal article or an abbreviated research report, you may not be in a position to make a judgement on these factors, but you do need to bear them in mind if you are thinking about implementing the findings from the study. For more details, see Gibbon (1995) or any in-depth text on research design.

There is one further point you need to be aware of – **bias**. This is a positive or negative influence on a concept, theory or attitude that is determined by errors in the research design, e.g. in the setting and wording of the research tools, in the sample selection or in the interpretation of data.

Some advantages and disadvantages of research tools are considered in the following sections. Think about whether or not these are relevant to the piece of research you are reading.

Questionnaires

Advantages	Disadvantages
Can be given to several people at the same time, e.g. to a whole class.	Takes time and effort to prepare and to test for reliability and validity (see above). May be expensive to print and reproduce.
Can be answered anonymously, therefore respondents may be more truthful.	Respondents may not be able to express their opinions or seek clarification.
May be easier for researcher to analyse and code responses.	Some people just do not like forms!
Respondents cannot be put off by the status of the researcher.	Respondents may complete their questionnaires casually, not bothering about their answers so as to get the questionnaire out of the way.

Advantages

Several people can answer at one time, so respondents' and researcher's time can be used more effectively.

Disadvantages

Respondents may give the answer that they think should be given, as if they were trying to supply the correct answer in a test, especially if the researcher is in some position of power or senior to them.

The researcher cannot ask a respondent to clarify answers.

- Were questionnaires used in the study you are reading?
- Was the questionnaire designed by the researcher?
- If so, how was its reliability and validity tested? In other words, is it reliable and does it measure what it is supposed to do?
- If you are familiar with the subject area of the research study (e.g. children in hospital), would you have asked those questions in relation to the aims of the study?
- Have important issues been missed by the questionnaire?
- Are the questions unambiguous? (If you are reading a journal the questions may not be given.)
- Are the questions suitably worded for respondents? For example, a questionnaire that asks mothers about their sick children must be worded differently from a questionnaire to doctors treating the same group of children.
- When were the questionnaires completed? Were the respondents tired or had they just been given bad or good news, etc? Does the researcher give you any indication of such facts?
- Were there any other significant factors that might have affected their answers?
- Did a group of respondents complete the questionnaires together so that they may have talked about their answers to produce a consensus opinion rather than individual views?

I am sure you can think of several other factors that affect not only the design of questionnaires but also how they are completed; how did the researcher try to ensure against these factors?

There are many articles reporting the use of questionnaires; these studies may be quantitative and/or qualitative, e.g. descriptive studies by Love (1996) and Laszlo and Strettle (1996) or an experimental study by Hicks (1996).

Interviews

Before setting out the advantages and disadvantages it is best to consider the different types of interview. In some cases it is essential that exactly the same questions are asked in exactly the same way, rather like a verbal questionnaire. This is a **structured interview**. A more flexible approach is gained from a **semi-structured interview** (e.g. Hicks *et al.*, 1996; Jerrett and Costello, 1996, where the researcher has some headings or points to be covered in the interview but not a strict format. An **unstructured interview** is what it sounds like. Apart from setting the topic it is more like a discourse between two people. The researcher does not guide the direction or flow of the interview.

Advantages	Disadvantages
The person being interviewed, the interviewee, can seek clarification and so can the researcher.	The researcher needs to be skilled in interview techniques.
The interviewee may be able to express views and opinions more easily verbally than in writing.	The interviewee may not like, or may be fearful of, the interviewer.
The researcher can check for misunderstandings due to culture or dialect. For example, in the UK, 'presently' means 'soon' or 'in a short while'; in the USA, however, 'presently' means 'now' or 'at the present'.	The interviewee may reply how he or she thinks she should do, in order to please the researcher or to appear in a good light.
In semi-structured or unstructured interviews, interesting lines of thought can be followed up and explored.	The interviewer can bias the interview, even unwittingly, by non-verbal cues, e.g. frowning at certain information so that the interviewee does not elaborate or mention it again. The reverse can also happen.
The interview may provide more flexibility for the researcher and interviewee. This depends on the design of the study.	Interviews are time-consuming.
	There may be difficulties in recording the information from the interview.
	There may be difficulties in analysing and coding the information.
	Interviews are not anonymous.

Use your experience and knowledge to think about the situations or topics where these three types of interview would be most appropriate.

- Were interviews used in the study you are reading?
- If they were used, which type was used and do you think it was the most suitable interview schedule?
- What could have been gained or lost through using a different format for the interviews?

(Note: the interview schedule is likely to be in the appendices of the full report.)

Participant observation

Recently reported studies using participant observation will provide you with an idea of how this research tool is used. Example, Clarke (1996) used participant observation in a secure unit, while Waterman *et al.* (1996) used participant observation as an opportunity to evaluate the introduction of case management in a rehabilitation unit for the elderly.

Advantages	Disadvantages
The researcher is part of the situation, so may be aware of less tangible aspects such as morale, apathy, goodwill.	The researcher may have difficulty in making objective observations if involved in the situation.
The researcher may be seen as having credibility by those being observed.	The researcher may have difficulty in recording observations, especially if working in a busy clinical area.
	The participants involved in the observations may see the researcher as a threat or spy, affecting the accuracy of observation.

Non-participant observation

Torrance and Serginson (1996) used non-participant techniques to assess the preparation of student nurses in the measurement of arterial blood pressure. Ragneskog *et al.* (1996) used video recording as part of a field experiment of the effect of different types of music at meal times on five patients suffering from dementia.

Advantages	Disadvantages
As the researcher is not involved in the situation, she/he may be able to make more objective observations.	The observer may be conspicuous, affecting what is being observed.
Researcher may be able to follow a plan of observation.	Two observers are often necessary to guard against observer bias, which takes time.
	There is a limit to the amount of time for which a researcher can observe.
	It is difficult to maintain objectivity at times.

This rather long chapter has considered some of the aspects you may encounter when you read how the research study was carried out and how the information or data was collected. I hope that some of the mystery has been taken out of this process and that your skills of enquiry and questioning have been stimulated. Now that you are aware of how the study was carried out, it is time to look at the results.

Answer to question on page 41.

Level of parental knowledge   the *independent variable*

Infants' sleep behaviour   the *dependent variable*.

8
The results

This section of the report is the one that many nurses find daunting, with tables, statistics and more unfamiliar terms. There is no room in this book to discuss all the terms you may encounter. Rather I will give you some advice that I hope will make the results section of any research piece easier to approach. I will also define a small number of the most common terms.

First, don't panic! You already know what the study is about, having read the summary and the conclusions. The results are what they say they are: findings on which the conclusions were based. However, it is important that you read the results in an informed way so that you can be sure the researcher is drawing reasonable conclusions from them. If the results show, for example, that there is a slight difference in management expertise between six medical ward sisters who had been in post two years compared with six medical sisters who had been in post five years, it would be unwise (given the small sample size and the slight difference) for the researcher to conclude that length of experience affected *all* ward sisters' management expertise.

Second, read carefully all titles or captions accompanying tables and figures. The unclear or overwhelming will soon start to make sense if you take the time to read what it says. Do not be baffled by the figures. *Stop*, *look* and *think*. Let that be your 'highway code' to guide you safely through the results section.

Third, if you still don't understand, get help. You need to be sure that you understand the essentials of the report. This is especially important if you are thinking of implementing the findings.

The following terms are well worth mastering as they are used frequently. Familiarity with them will help you to understand what you are reading.

Mean

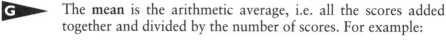

The **mean** is the arithmetic average, i.e. all the scores added together and divided by the number of scores. For example:

$$5 + 3 + 2 + 6 + 6 + 1 + 5 + 6 + 1 + 4 + 5 + 6 + 1 + 6 + 3 = 60$$

Therefore, the mean is $60/15 = 4$.

Median

The **median** is the number that occurs in the middle of an ordered sequence of scores. For example, if the above scores are rearranged as

$$1 + 1 + 1 + 2 + 3 + 3 + 4 + 5 + 5 + 5 + 6 + 6 + 6 + 6 + 6 = 60$$

the median is 5.

Mode

The **mode** is the score that occurs most frequently in a range of scores. In the above example, the score 6 occurs five times. Therefore, the mode is 6.

You can see how exactly the same scores provide a different answer depending on which arithmetical 'treatment' is used, so be careful in your reading.

> Here is a little story that may help you see the relevance of each term. I had the pleasure of knowing a wonderful 82-year-old lady from Scotland. She suffered from angina, which was aggravated by the cold. Her flat faced north and was very cold in winter. But being a true Scot she was very economical. As soon as her daughter had gone to work she turned the heating off, or right down, and did not turn it up again until just before her daughter was due home! The evenings were therefore quite cosy and warm. If the temperature of the flat had been recorded every hour during the day and the *mean* (the average temperature) used as a measure

of her living environment, it would probably have been above the level to worry about hypothermia. However, if readings had been taken hourly throughout the day and ranked in ascending order, the *median* (the reading in the middle of the sequence) would have given a truer picture. If the *mode* (the most frequent reading) had been used, this might have revealed a worrying but accurate picture because the temperature of the flat would have been low on six or seven occasions during the day. This information could have been clearly seen if the temperatures had been plotted on a graph.

■ In your own work, when would each of these three terms be of most use to you? Make a note of your examples.

Presenting data visually

You are familiar with graphs, especially in the form of temperature charts. However, there are a number of points concerning the interpretation of graphical material that might cause you problems.

I have already highlighted the importance of reading the captions that accompany any table, graph, pie or bar chart. The titles or captions inform you about the information (data) that you are about to consider. If you are confronted with a graph or a bar chart, read the title carefully and look at the numerical ranges of both the horizontal and vertical axes.

Graphs

Figure 8.1 shows a patient's temperature chart. The caption would show the patient's name, the name of the ward or unit and whether the temperature was recorded four-hourly or daily. The horizontal axis gives the date and time and the vertical axis is marked off in degrees Celsius.

In reality many temperature charts are three graphs one above the other, showing temperature, pulse and respiration (TPR). Each graph shares the same horizontal information (date and time) but the vertical axes for each graph are different and have different numerical ranges to reflect the nature of the recordings. For instance, in Fig. 8.1 the vertical axis for temperature ranges from 35 to 41°C; each degree is subdivided into tenths so that a patient's temperature can be recorded as, for example, 37.4°C. However, the vertical axis for pulse rate is

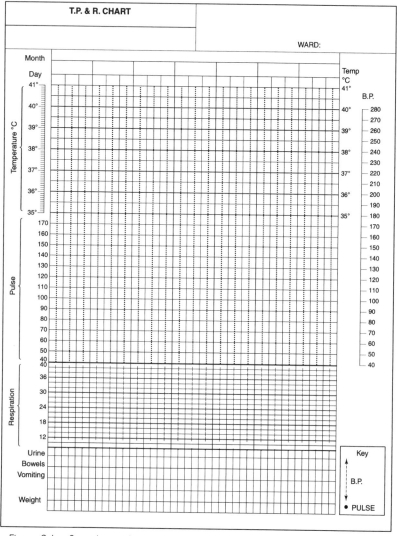

Figure 8.1   Sample graph: a patient's temperature chart.

numbered from 40 to 170 divided into tens (i.e. 40, 50, 60, etc.); each division of 10 is subdivided into fifths so that the smallest division equals two. The vertical axis for respiratory rate is numbered from 12 to 40 divided into sixes (i.e. 12, 18, 24, etc.); each division of six is subdivided into thirds so that the smallest division is again two.

Most of you complete and/or read TPR charts accurately and with little hesitation, so remember these skills and transfer them to your appraisal of other graphs you may encounter in the report you are reading.

Figure 8.2 is taken from a study of the influence of music on the feeding and eating behaviour of patients suffering from dementia (Ragneskog *et al.*, 1996). What can you learn from a look at this graph? The graph shows the time (in minutes) five patients spent with their dinner under four conditions, three with different types of music and one control period. The graph shows at a glance that there was variation between patients and slight variation between conditions.

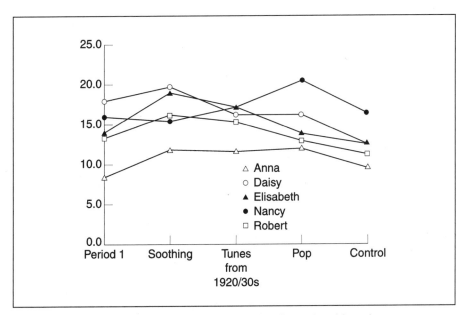

Figure 8.2   Sample graph: time spent on dinner. (From Ragneskog, H. et al. (1996) Clinical Nursing Research 5, 262–282. With permission of Sage Publications.)

Pie charts

A pie chart resembles a pie divided into slices. The slices represent the size of a particular category; the larger the slice the larger that particular category. For example, Fig. 8.3a represents the numbers of Christmas cards I usually send to different locations. The smallest slice indicates those that are sent overseas, the medium-sized slice those delivered locally and the largest slice those delivered within the UK. I could also choose to consider how many cards were sent to businesses, service providers, family and friends, and this would produce a different pie chart (Fig. 8.3b).

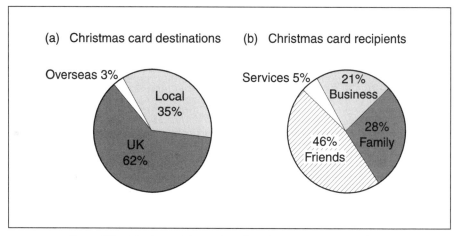

Figure 8.3   Pie charts: (a) number of cards sent by location; (b) number of cards sent by type of recipient.

Bar charts

However, if I wished to see how the above distribution had changed over time it would be easier to use a bar chart (Fig. 8.4). As with graphs, look carefully at the captions and the frequency/distribution ranges along the axes.

Examine the bar chart in Fig. 8.5, taken from a journal article about how nurse teachers keep up to date (Love, 1996). From this chart it is possible to see at a glance which of the activities was regarded as indispensable by the nurse teachers for keeping up to date.

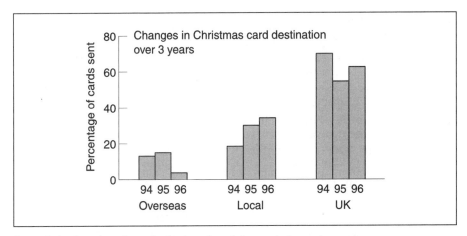

Figure 8.4   Bar chart: how distribution of cards has varied over three years.

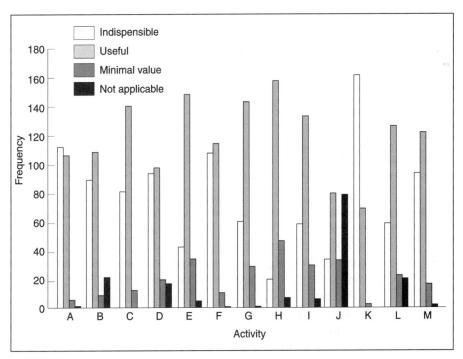

Figure 8.5   Bar chart: how nurse teachers keep up to date. (From Love, C. 1996) Nurse Education Today **16**, 287–295. With permission of Churchill Livingstone.)

■ Which activity was regarded as indispensable by nurse teachers?
See page 64 for answer.

From studying these examples I hope you feel more comfortable when looking at charts, graphs and figures and realize that they are simply a way of presenting data in a more interesting way that enables you to see similarities, differences, spreads and trends at a glance. Therefore, take your time and read carefully any figures or graphs in the report you are reading.

If you still feel unhappy about interpreting data, Hicks (1994) is a clear straightforward article that covers the route from tabulated data to the presentation of that data in various graphical forms; it is well worth reading.

Some terms that are frequently used in the results section of reports are now examined.

Significance (significance level, statistical significance)

We use the word 'significant' in our everyday conversations, perhaps to tell our friends about a significant point in our lives; in other words, when something memorable happened to us that may have altered the course of our lives, like getting our first job or getting married.

In research the word 'significance' has a specific and rather precise use. It refers to **statistical significance**. When a piece of research has been carried out, especially if an experimental design was used (as in Boore, 1978 and Kerr *et al.*, 1996, both discussed earlier), the researcher wants to be sure that the findings did not occur due to chance or to one or two extreme cases. In other words, how *probable* is it that the information given to the experimental group is low for post-operative stress or better sleep in infants is really due to the independent variable, rather than a chance happening?

Probability (P) is another term frequently used in reports and is closely linked to significance. Probability is a measure of whether an event is likely to occur. By convention, probability is measured from one (the event is inevitable) to zero (the event is impossible). In life most events are somewhere in the middle. If you would like to read more, Harris (1986) provides a readable account of these issues.

Tests of significance

Having introduced these two terms, we now proceed to think about how the researcher attempts to verify that the results obtained were not due to chance. We can never be sure whether results are due to chance or not, but we can work out the probability that they might be due to chance; this is **statistical inference**. There are many statistical tests available, and different tests are appropriate in different conditions and situations. The choice of test is beyond the scope of this book. You will not be in a position to question whether the correct test was used. However, as you are likely to be reading published research you may assume that a panel of knowledgeable experts will have vetted the report before it was published.

Tests of significance indicate whether the difference between the *observed* results and those *expected* from the original hypothesis is likely to have been due to chance. The **level of significance** is derived from statistical tests, the results of which are compared with statistical tables (which can be found in any statistical textbook, along with instructions to work out the test).

Chi-squared test

One of the commonly used tests of significance in many nursing research reports is the **chi-squared (χ^2) test**. The chi-squared test is used on datasets that are organized into categories rather than scores.

The example below is taken from Atkinson and Sklaroff (1987). In chapter 4 of their monograph there are several statements similar to the one below:

$$\chi^2 = 19.884, 4\text{df}, P < 0.001$$

where < means less than and > means greater than. The abbreviation 'df' refers to **degrees of freedom**, which is calculated as part of the statistical test and is used to determine the level of significance. The chi-squared (χ^2) value obtained from the results of the research in the example above is compared with figures in a table of probabilities at the 4df level.

In the context of tests of significance, probability refers to the likelihood of the experimental results differing from those expected from the original hypothesis by random chance. The nearer the value of P to zero, the smaller the likelihood that the difference between observed and expected data is due to chance and, therefore, the more significant the experimental findings.

There are accepted guidelines for assessing the significance of the difference between the observed and the expected data. When $P < 0.05$ (e.g. 0.04, 0.03, 0.02), the difference is said to be *significant*. For $P > 0.05$ (e.g. 0.06, 0.08, 0.1), the difference is said to be not significant (NS). When P is much less than 0.05, the difference between the observed and expected data assumes a greater level of significance. At $P < 0.01$ and $P < 0.001$ the differences by convention attain significance of higher orders of magnitude. Sometimes a probability value for a chi-squared test will be followed by one, two or three asterisks, denoting probabilities of less than 0.05, 0.01 and 0.001 respectively.

t-Test

Another commonly used statistical test of significance is the *t*-test. The chi-squared test is a test of significance between datasets organized into categories, e.g. helpers and non-helpers, whereas the *t*-test is a significance test for the difference between two sets of scores.

Some of the research studies already mentioned have used these tests. For instance, Hicks (1996) gives the results of a *t*-test on characteristics related to the gender of researchers, while Clement *et al.* (1996) used a chi-squared test to examine women's satisfaction with antenatal care and the variables that might influence satisfaction with altered frequency of visits.

Distribution

We have seen that the mean is a useful statistic. When considered with other statistics such as the median and the mode, an idea of the **distribution** of a number of observations may be obtained. A better measure of such distribution is the **standard deviation**. This statistic is calculated from the amount by which each score differs from the mean of all scores. For example, in a test a group of seven student nurses (Group 1)

are given marks out of 10. If the scores are 9, 1, 2, 4, 8, 5 and 6, the mean is 5 but the scores range from 9 to 1; this indicates a wide range in their knowledge. However, if another group of seven student nurses (Group 2) sitting the same test score 6, 4, 4, 5, 5, 6 and 5, the mean is the same as Group 1 (i.e. 5) but the variation in the scores is much smaller (from 4 to 6). In this example the standard deviation for the scores differs, being higher in Group 1 where the range of scores is greater. (For further information on the calculation and interpretation of standard deviation see Reid and Boore, 1987 or Couchman and Dawson, 1995.) If you are reading a report that gives the result as a mean score, look at the size of the standard deviation; it could be very important. In the example above, you cannot assume that a group mean of 5, half the possible marks, demonstrates that all the students are reasonably proficient. First, *stop*, *look* and *think*. In Group 1, which had the higher standard deviation, one student scored only 1 and another 2. These scores do not indicate proficiency. Yet Group 2, with the same mean, might be considered a reasonably proficient group as two students were only one mark below the mean. I am sure you can think of examples in your work where a wide range of results could be very important.

Correlation

The final term discussed in this section is the **coefficient of correlation**. This is a numerical index used to indicate the degree of correspondence (match) between two sets of measurements, e.g. the degree of agreement between two nurses rating the behaviour of a hyperactive child or two nurses rating the size of varicose ulcers.

A coefficient of correlation of 1 indicates a perfect match (i.e. a one-to-one agreement); 0.9 indicates a near perfect match or *correlation*; 0.5 indicates only half agreement and 0.2 virtually no match or correlation; −1.0 indicates a perfect negative correlation.

There are various statistical tests used to calculate the coefficient of correlation, which are described in more detail in Reid and Boore (1987) or Couchman and Dawson (1995). Remember, the nearer to 1, the better the correlation.

Summary

I hope you find these brief descriptions useful when making your way through the results section in the research report you are reading. Remember to complete your summary sheet.

Remember that at the back of this book is the Glossary, which defines the terms considered here. As you read more reports, you might find it helpful to compile your own dictionary of terms.

Having considered the most factual part of the report we now move on to consider how the researcher interprets the results in light of the aim of the study and other relevant factors.

Answer to question on page 60 is Activity K which was reading journals.

9
The discussion and conclusion

Key words:
- Review
- Summary
- References
- Appendices

In the last two chapters you encountered many new terms. There are no new terms in this chapter, which looks at the last parts of a research report, the *discussion* and *conclusion*. The discussion contains an analysis of the results and a **review** of the study as a whole. The conclusion is a **summary** of the whole study. While reading the discussion of your chosen report you need to use your nursing knowledge and expertise, as well as common sense, in order to consider the veracity of the arguments made by the researcher.

Discussion

In this part of a research report the researcher discusses the results given in the previous section and relates them to the initial research question. The results will also be considered in relation to the work reviewed in the literature search and to any other relevant aspects (e.g. clinical applications).

Turn to your summary sheet and remind yourself about the aim of the study. If you have not yet summarized the results onto the summary sheet, do so now. Writing this summary will help you to clarify your thoughts and focus on pertinent points. Now that you have done this, there are some questions you should bear in mind as you read the discussion.

■ Would you make the same inferences as the researcher does from what you have just read?
■ How do the results of the present study support/contradict previous work?
■ What are the limitations of the study? For example, is the study limited by sample size (consult your summary sheet)? Is the study limited by its specificity or can some findings be more widely applied (e.g. does a piece of research on weight gain in premature babies have any implications for the care of other babies)?
■ What implications can be drawn from the research?

Conclusion

This final part of the report summarizes all that has gone before. Usually, it also points the way forward to further research and/or application of the findings.

■ What has this piece of research added to the body of knowledge?
■ How could or should it affect nursing care, policy or procedure?
■ Even if the research was not carried out in your speciality, what are the implications for your area? An example of the implications of one research study being applied to a different situation can be seen in Pat Ashworth's (1980) study. This piece of research was carried out among intensive care nurses, yet the findings, about how nurses communicate or fail to communicate with patients unable to respond, has been found to be most helpful in relation to care of the elderly.
■ What have you learned from the research about (a) the topic being researched and (b) the research process?

Now summarize the conclusion onto the summary sheet. This completes the first side of the summary sheet; the reverse side can be used to discuss how the findings could be applied in your area of nursing. (I discuss the application of research findings in Chapter 10.)

You have reached the end of the main part of the research report. The remainder of the report contains the **references**, the sources for all the material referred to during the report. If you have been reading a research report rather than a journal article there may also be **appendices** and a **bibliography**. It is likely that you will have consulted the appendices while you were looking at questionnaire items and/or the interview schedule.

At this point you should complete the index card you prepared at the start. Summarize the main points of the research report, giving just enough detail for it to make sense to you in six months' time. I suggest that as you complete these cards you keep a record of the subject codes you choose, as it will be difficult to remember what they stand for after a few weeks or months.

With your finished report, your completed card, your notes and (I hope) your new-found confidence, this is an appropriate moment for a little reflection.

- What was your aim when you started reading the research report?
- Was it part of a course requirement or did someone else say you should read it?
- Do you understand what you have read?

If you still have doubts, I include some more detailed texts that explain more fully some of the topics that could only be mentioned briefly in this introductory book. It may be that you will need to look at the study in more depth or obtain a copy of the full report or thesis, in which case your local librarian will probably be able to help. Alternatively, a discussion with a colleague may help to clarify your ideas.

In the final chapter, I consider the implications of research for practice.

10
Implications for practice

Key words:
- Research-based profession
- Evidence-based practice
- Implementation

We looked at some of the issues related to why research is important in relation to **research-based profession** and **evidence-based practice** in the first two chapters. Having read your piece of research with the aid of this book, you need to ask yourself: Has the research report any use or relevance for everyday work?

At the start of this book we examined the research related to pressure areas that was carried out by Doreen Norton 35 years ago and the subsequent research and clinical practice, only to find that ritual, non-research-based treatments are still being carried out. Sadly, Tross (1995), reviewing the care of wounds and pressure sores, reports that research-based care is not prevalent. She concludes:

> 'If nurses are to be encouraged to apply research findings to the care of wounds and pressure sores, it is important for related policies and procedures to reflect such findings. Nurses must also be encouraged to consult the references provided and to review them with a critical eye, with a view to ensuring that wound care management is in line with current thinking and knowledge of the subject.' (p. 28)

Professor Tony Butterworth (1994) describes the long process (36 years) of a research idea with abstract theoretical beginnings that turned into an everyday practice activity. He describes psychosocial interventions with people with schizophrenia, outlining four phases and the policy matters, educational changes, service provision and various other influences on the development of the process. He concludes that research has no clear end-point, but the importance of persevering with a research idea cannot be overestimated. I would add that this applies equally to the reading and understanding of research.

The Report of the Committee on Nursing (Briggs Report) (Department of Health and Social Security, 1972) urged that nursing should become a research-based profession; over 20 years later the UK government is embracing the idea of evidence-based practice. Deighan and Boyd (1996) studied the origins of the concept of evidence-based practice and concluded that it should extend to all aspects of the NHS not just clinical work. Evidence-based health care derives from the term 'evidence-based medicine', which was seen as a learning strategy for clinical medicine in Canada in the 1980s. Deighan and Boyd (1996) provide two definitions, written about medicine but which could easily apply to nursing.

> 'Sackett *et al.* provide a comprehensive definition of evidence-based medicine, describing it as follows: "The practice of evidence-based medicine is therefore an integration of individual clinical expertise with the best available external clinical evidence from systematic research". Rosenberg and Donald provide a different angle to the practice of evidence-based medicine, describing it as "a process of turning clinical problems into questions and then systematically locating, appraising and using contemporaneous research findings as the basis for clinical decisions".' (p. 333)

So, how are you going to assess the relevance of the report you have just read and address the persistent call for care to be research based? To a certain extent, you are already well on the way to answering this question by having tackled a report and read this book. The following questions may help you consider how the research findings can best be applied to nursing practice.

- Are you sure the findings are valid and reliable?
- Are there other studies or reports to support the findings?
- Are there other studies or reports to contradict the findings?
- You will find the references at the end of the report you have been reading useful in helping you answer the last two questions. Remember, however, that the references indicate research that was written *before* the research you are reading; you may need to conduct a literature search for more recent material.

- If you have read a summary of the research and think that it is useful to you and that the findings could be implemented, have you read the original source in order to look at all the limitations and pitfalls?
- How practical will it be to implement the findings? Look at both the costs and benefits. List them. Don't forget the hidden costs such as training time for new techniques, increased anxiety at a time of change, etc.
- Who would be involved in the implementation, both directly and indirectly? Don't forget issues related to the storage and disposal of equipment, porterage, unions, staff training and continuing education departments.

When you have listed all these, stop, look and think again.

- Why should there be change?
- Is the contemplated change for the better?

If after you have answered all these questions you still think that implementation of the research findings is a good idea, approach your line manager with a succinct summary of the research, including a copy of your summary sheet, the answers to the above questions, together with a list of advantages and disadvantages of implementation. This will make your argument more balanced from the start. Sooner or later, someone is bound to point out the contradictions, cost, implications and potential problems, so that person might as well be you. In this way you will be able to follow up with effective counter-arguments.

I hope that now you feel encouraged to read research and to use the knowledge you gain in this way. I hope that you read with purpose and that as you master the terms and concepts of the research process you will question not only what you read but also your own practices. Such questioning is essential to the pursuit of excellence. Research is not an alien thing; it *can* affect everyday nursing. You do not need to undertake research yourself to examine the findings that other people present and to consider whether and how they apply to your work. In the words of Baroness McFarlane of Llandaff (1984):

'Research is thus not a luxury for the academic, but a tool for developing the quality of nursing decisions, prescriptions and action. Whether as clinicians, educators, managers or researchers we have a research responsibility; neglect of that responsibility could be classed as professional negligence.'

In June 1996, the Foundation of Nursing Studies published *Reflection for Action: Putting Research into Practice*. The Foundation's aim is to 'disseminate, use and implement proven research findings to improve patient care'. Mulhall (1996) writing about the background to the organization states:

'Research is used when it is accessed, read and evaluated with a view to increasing knowledge and understanding. Implementation occurs when changes, based on the results of research are made in practice. These activities rely not only on the availability of relevant research, but more crucially on the critical evaluation of that knowledge.'

She goes on to say how important it is that research findings are translated into the language and action of practice and that there is an opportunity to sustain change based on research findings. I hope that you will contribute to the application of research using the knowledge you have gained while reading this book.

Take heart – you are not alone. There may be a journal club in your unit or locality, or you may find there is a local research interest group. These will give you support, allow you to share interests and to form a body of research-based information.

Do you feel inspired to go on and read some more? At the very least I hope you are feeling more positive about nursing research and more ready to consider the ways in which research findings may be positively applied to improve your practice. Lathlean (1988) describes how clinical nurses have applied research findings to their work areas and altered various aspects of their practice, so it *can* be done. Now that you have made a summary of one piece of research and completed a record card, I hope you feel prepared and ready to tackle some more research reports.

Finally, the Further reading and Reference sections provide you with books and articles that you may find useful as you continue your research reading.

References

Ashworth, P. (1980) *Care to Communicate. An Investigation into the Problems of Communication between Patients and Nurses in Intensive Therapy Units.* London: Royal College of Nursing.

Astbury, C. (1988) *Stress and the Nurse in the Operating Theatre.* London: Royal College of Nursing.

Atkinson, F. I. & Sklaroff, S. A. (1987) *Acute Hospital Wards and the Disabled Patient. A Survey of the Experiences of Patients and Nurses.* London: Royal College of Nursing.

Ballie, L. (1995) Ethnography and nursing research: a critical appraisal. *Nurse Researcher* 3, 5–21.

Barrett, M. C., Arklie, M. M. & Smillie, C. (1996) Evaluating the graduates of the Dalhousie University School of Nursing baccalaureate programme: a quantitative/qualitative responsive model. *Journal of Advanced Nursing* 24, 1070–1076.

Boore, J. R. P. (1978) *Prescription for Recovery. The Effect of Pre-operative Preparation of Surgical Patients on Post-operative Stress, Recovery and Infection.* London: Royal College of Nursing.

Bradshaw, A. (1994) *Lighting the Lamp. The Spiritual Dimension of Nursing Care.* London: Royal College of Nursing.

Brazier, H. & Begley, C. M. (1996) Selecting a database for literature searches in nursing: MEDLINE or CINAHL. *Journal of Advanced Nursing* 24, 868–875.

Bromley, P. (1986) A sore point with nurses. *Nursing Times* 82(32), 65.

Butterworth, T. (1994) Developing research ideas: from theory to practice. *Nurse Researcher* 14, 78–86.

Clarke, L. (1996) Participant observation in a secure unit: care, conflict and control. *NTResearch* 1, 431–441.

Clement, S., Sikorski, J., Wilson, J., Das, S. & Smeeton, N. (1996) Women's satisfaction with traditional and reduced antenatal visit schedules. *Midwifery* 12, 120–128.

Coates, V. (1985) *Are They Being Served? An Investigation into the Nutritional Care given by Nurses to Acute Medical Patients and the Influence of Ward Organisational Patterns of Care.* London: Royal College of Nursing.

Cortis, J. D. & Lacey, A. E. (1996) Measuring quality and quantity of information-giving to in-patients. *Journal of Advanced Nursing* 24, 674–681.

Couchman, W. & Dawson, J. (1995) *Nursing and Health-Care Research. A Practical Guide.* London: Scutari Press.

Deacon, L. (1986) Does anyone read research? *Nursing Times* 82(32), 58–59.

Deighan, M. & Boyd, K. (1996). Defining evidenced-based health care: a health-care strategy? *NTResearch* 1, 332–338.

Department of Health (1993) *Report of the Taskforce on the Strategy for Research in Nursing, Midwifery and Health Visiting*, Annexes 1–4. London: Royal College of Nursing.

Department of Health (1994) *Supporting Research and Development in the National Health Service*. The Culyer Report. London: HMSO.

Department of Health and Social Security, Scottish Home and Health Department and Welsh Office (1972) *Report of the Committee on Nursing*. The Briggs Report. London: HMSO.

Department of Health and Social Security. Nursing Research Abstracts. London, DHSS.

De Raeve, L. (ed.) (1996) *Nursing Research: An Ethical and Legal Appraisal*. London: Baillière Tindall.

Dubyna, J. & Quinn, C. (1996) The self-management of psychiatric medications: a pilot study. *Journal of Psychiatric and Mental Health Nursing* 3, 297–302.

East, I. & Robinson, J. (1994) Change in process: bringing about change in health care through action research. *Journal of Clinical Nursing* 3, 57–61.

Edmonstone, J. (1996) Strengthening cancer care: a practical approach to the empowerment of nurses. *NTResearch* 15, 382–388.

Faulkner, A. (1984) *Teaching non-specialist nurses assessment skills in the aftercare of mastectomy patients*. PhD Thesis, University of Manchester.

Foundation of Nursing Studies (1996) *Putting Research into Practice: Reflection for Action*. London: Foundation of Nursing Studies.

Franklin, B. L. (1974) *Patient Anxiety on Admission to Hospital*. London: Royal College of Nursing.

Fretwell, J. E. (1982) *Ward Teaching and Learning: Sister and the Learning Environment*. London: Royal College of Nursing.

Fretwell, J. E. (1985) *Freedom to Change. The Creation of a Ward Learning Environment*. London: Royal College of Nursing.

Gibbon, B. (1995) Validity and reliability of assessment tools. *Nurse Researcher* 2, 48–55.

Gott, M. (1984) *Learning Nursing*. London: Royal College of Nursing.

Grahn, G. & Danielson, M. (1996) Coping with the cancer experience. II Evaluating an education and support programme for cancer patients and their significant others. *European Journal of Cancer Care* 5, 182–187.

Hallett, C. (1995) Understanding the phenomenological approach to research. *Nurse Researcher* 3, 55–65.

Harris, P. (1986) *Designing and Reporting Experiments*. Milton Keynes: Open University Press.

Henderson, V. (1987) *Clinical Excellence in Nursing: International Networking*. Indianapolis: Sigma Theta Tau International.

Hicks, C. (1994) Using tables and graphs to present research findings. *Nurse Researcher* 2, 54–74.

Hicks, C. (1996) The potential impact of gender stereotypes for nursing research. *Journal of Advanced Nursing* 24, 1006–1013.

Hicks, C., Hennessy, D., Cooper, J. & Barwell, F. (1996) Investigating attitudes to research in primary health care teams. *Journal of Advanced Nursing* 24, 1033–1041.

Hulland, S. M. (1985) *A comparison of nurses' actions and beliefs in relation to pressure sore prophylaxis and treatment*. MSc Thesis, University of Manchester.

Isles, J. (1986) An eradication campaign. *Nursing Times* 82(32), 59–62.

Jerrett, M. D. & Costello, E. A. (1996) Gaining control: parents' experiences of accommodating children's asthma. *Clinical Nursing Research* 5, 294–308.

Kerr, S. M., Jowett, S. A. & Smith, L. N. (1996) Preventing sleep problems in infants: a randomized controlled trial. *Journal of Advanced Nursing* 24, 938–942.

Kirkevold, M., Berg, K. & Saltvold, S. (1996) Patterns of recovery among Norwegian heart surgery patients. *Journal of Advanced Nursing* 24, 943–951.

Laszlo, H. & Strettle, R. (1996) Midwives' motivation for continuing education. *Nurse Education Today* 16, 363–367.

Lathlean, J. (1988) *Research in Action: Developing the Role of the Ward Sister*. London: Kings Fund Centre.

Love, C. (1996) How nurse teachers keep up-to-date: their methods and practices. *Nurse Education Today* 16, 287–295.

McFarlane of Llandaff (1984) The future. In *The Research Process in Nursing*, ed. Cormack, D. F. S. p. x. Oxford: Blackwell Scientific Publications.

McGonagle, I. M. & Gentle, J. (1996) Reasons for non-attendance at a day hospital for people with enduring mental illness: the clients' perspective. *Journal of Psychiatric and Mental Health Nursing* 3, 1–66.

Mead, D. (1996) Teaching nursing and midwifery research. In *Nursing Research: An Ethical and Legal Appraisal*, ed. De Raeve, L. pp. 160–182. London: Baillière Tindall.

Moorbath, P. (1995) Libraries for nursing/RCN survey on access to libraries for qualified nurses. *Libraries for Nursing Bulletin* 15, 13–31.

Moores, Y. (1996) The research agenda: change, challenge, opportunity. *NTResearch* 1, 330–331.

Mulhall, A. (1996) Background to *Putting Research into Practice: Reflection for Action*. London: Foundation of Nursing Studies.

Newton, C. A. (1995) Action research: application in practice. *Nurse Researcher* 2, 60–71.

Norton, D., McLaren, R. & Exton-Smith, N. (1962) *An Investigation of Geriatric Nursing Problems in Hospital*. Edinburgh: Churchill Livingstone.

Ogier, M. E. (1982) *An Ideal Sister?* London: Royal College of Nursing.

Powell, D. (1982) *Learning to Relate?* London: Royal College of Nursing.

Ragneskog, H., Kihlgren, M., Karlsson, I. & Norberg, A. (1996) Dinner music for demented patients: analysis of video-recorded observations. *Clinical Nursing Research* 5, 262–282.

Reid, N. G. & Boore, J. R. P. (1987) *Research Methods and Statistics in Health Care*. London: Edward Arnold.

Royal College of Nursing Nursing Bibliography. London, Royal College of Nursing.

Runciman, P., Currie, C. T., Nicol, M. & McKay, V. (1996) Discharge of elderly people from an accident and emergency department: evaluation of health visitor follow-up. *Journal of Advanced Nursing* **24**, 711–718.

Russell, C. K. & Gregory, D. M. (1993) Issues for consideration when choosing a qualitative data management system. *Journal of Advanced Nursing* **18**, 1806–1816.

Savage, J. (1995) *Nursing Intimacy: An Ethnographic Approach to Nurse–Patient Interaction.* London: Scutari Press.

Scottish Office Home and Health Department (1993) *Research and Development Strategy for the National Health Service in Scotland.* Edinburgh: HMSO.

Sleep, J. (1988) Reported in *Advances in Midwifery Research. Senior Nurse* **8**, 5.

Spouse, J. (1990) *An Ethos for Learning.* London: Scutari Press.

Stodulski, A. H. (1995) *Royal College of Nursing Study of UK Nursing Journals.* London: RCN Library Information Services.

Stonehouse, J. & Butcher, J. (1996) Phlebitis associated with peripheral cannulae. *Professional Nurse* **12**, 51–54.

Torrance, C. & Serginson, E. (1996) An observational study of student nurses' measurement of arterial blood pressure by sphygmomanometry and auscultation. *Nurse Education Today* **16**, 282–286.

Tross, G. (1995) Raising the issues. *Journal of Community Nursing* **9**, 26–28.

Twomey, M. (1987) Coping with mastectomy. *Senior Nurse* **7**, 10–11.

United Kingdom Central Council for Nursing, Midwifery and Health Visiting (1992) *Code of Professional Conduct for the Nurse, Midwife and Health Visitor*, 3rd edn. London: UKCC.

Waterman, H. (1995) Distinguishing between 'traditional' and action research. *Nurse Researcher* **2**, 15–23.

Waterman, H., Waters, K. & Awenat, Y. (1996) The introduction of case management on a rehabilitation floor. *Journal of Advanced Nursing* **24**, 960–967.

West, B. J. (1992) Action research and standards of care. The prevention and treatment of pressure sores in the elderly. *Scottish Health Bulletin* **6**, 356–361.

Further reading

Where to start

Powers, B. A. & Knapp, T. R. (1990) *A Dictionary of Nursing Theory and Research*. London: Sage Publications. A dictionary, but some of the definitions amount to explanations of several pages. A really useful book to have if you are a novice to research.

Clamp, C. G. L. & Gough, S. (1999) *Resources for Nursing Research: An Annotated Bibliography* 3rd edn. London: Sage Publications. This brings together literature relating to all aspects of research. It has breadth rather than depth, gives UK and North American references and has 1300 entries 95% of which are annotated. It is divided into three sections: research text, ethical issues on research, and teaching on nursing research.

Texts about research

I strongly recommend the following books as a follow-up to this book.

Couchman, W. & Dawson, J. (1995) *Nursing and Health-care Research. A Practical Guide*. London: Scutari Press (reprinted 1996 by Baillière Tindall). The authors write that the book operates at two levels: research appreciation and beginning actual research. I think you will find it very helpful: there are plenty of examples, exercises to help you assess your progress and understanding, and it is well referenced with suggestions for further reading.

Buckeldee, J. & McMahon, R. (1994) *The Research Experience in Nursing*. London: Chapman & Hall. Includes chapters on defining the research question, choosing a methodology, piloting a study, conducting interviews and making sense of data.

Cormack, D. F. S. (ed.) (1991) *The Research Process in Nursing*, 2nd edn. Oxford: Blackwell Scientific Publications. Many students find this text helpful.

The British Psychological Society has published four Open Learning Units on research design and statistics. These are aimed at A-level students studying psychology so you will not find any nursing examples, but they are easily understandable with plenty of everyday examples and some entertaining cartoons. They have the bonus of being cheap at £3.50 or £4.50 each.

- Unit 1: Models and Methods for the Behavioural Sciences
- Unit 2: Describing and Interpreting Data
- Unit 3: Drawing Inferences from Statistical Data

These three units were published in 1994. The fourth unit (Ethics in Psychological Research and Practice) was published in 1991. You are likely to find these units in any library that is not purely a nursing library.

Waltz, C. F., Strickland, O. L. & Lenz, E. R. (1984) *Measurements in Nursing Research*. Philadelphia: F. A. Davis. A very detailed and expensive book; library use!

Qualitative research

Field, P. A. & Morse, J. M. (1985) *Nursing Research: The Application of Qualitative Approaches*. London: Croom Helm (reprinted by Chapman & Hall).

Morse, J. M. (ed.) (1992) *Qualitative Health Research*. London: Sage Publications. Contains chapters on topics such as phenomenology, ethnomethodology, grounded theory, etc.

Bannister, P., Burman, E., Parker, I., Taylor, M. & Tindall, C. (1994) *Qualitative Methods in Psychology: A Research Guide*. Buckingham: Open University Press. A more advanced text on qualitative research methods.

Ethics and research

An important area that must be considered when reading and especially if considering carrying out research is ethics. To many the term 'ethics' is nearly as daunting as the word 'research'.

De Raeve, L. (ed.) (1996) *Nursing Research: An Ethical and Legal Appraisal*. London: Baillière Tindall. Louise de Raeve has collected contributions from 12 authors on various topics related to ethics and nursing; you will find them interesting and thoroughly grounded in nursing. An essential read for any nurse.

See also British Psychological Society and Clamp *et al.* (1991).

Statistics

Reid, N. G. & Boore, J. R. P. (1987) *Research Methods and Statistics in Health Care*. London: Edward Arnold. This book is well related to nursing practice, is written in a readable way and the statistics are carefully explained with worked examples.

Hicks, C. M. (1990) *Research and Statistics: A Practical Introduction for Nurses*. London: Prentice Hall. A useful, easily followed text.

Journals

Since the first edition was published there seems to have been a proliferation of nursing journals. I am extremely grateful to Ann Stodulski (formerly Librarian at the Royal College of Nursing) for a report she compiled on UK nursing journals, *Royal College of Nursing Study of UK Nursing Journals*. Should you want your own copy it is obtainable from the RCN Library Information Services price £15. If you have been asked to look at research on a particular topic, then a computer search will provide information quickly. However, there is a lag of about six months before references are included on the database, so for the most recent work you will need to turn to journals. In 1995, journals listed below were identified as featuring research reports on a regular basis:

- *Journal of Advanced Nursing*
- *Intensive and Critical Care Nursing*
- *International Journal of Nursing Studies*
- *Journal of Psychiatric and Mental Health Nursing*
- *Midwifery*
- *Nurse Education Today*
- *Nurse Researcher.*

You may find help with understanding the research process by looking at specific issues of *Nurse Researcher*, a journal of research methodology published quarterly. It is aimed at pre- and post-registration students and nurses in practice and education, with papers on research methods related to useful examples of clinical practice. Each issue has a specific theme, e.g. sampling, interviewing, observational studies, action research, ethnography and phenomenology. Volume 1, no. 1 was published in September 1993 and over the years a useful collection of papers and ideas have accrued.

Even since Ann Stodulski produced her report in 1995, other journals have appeared and, with the push for a research-based practice, more and more journals are increasing their research content. For instance, *NTResearch* is a bimonthly journal that aims to publish research on nursing topics and themes; unfortunately, the references are in very small print at present. Each month during 1995, the *Journal of Community Nursing* included an article on the research process.

There are other nursing research journals that are produced outside the UK. I have used at least two references from *Clinical Nursing Research*, an international journal produced in Canada that publishes refereed articles which focus on clinical practice.

Actual research reports

The Royal College of Nursing used to publish completed doctoral and masters theses in abbreviated form, which were accessible and easily readable. The last one was published in 1994.

In 1974, the Steinberg Collection of theses and dissertations, either by nurses or on topics related to nursing in the UK, was set up and is housed in the Royal College of Nursing. In 1995, there were 724 items from 128 universities in the collection. You are able to obtain these on loan only through university libraries or from the British Library Document Supply Centre. A catalogue is available. However, may I suggest that this is not your first line of enquiry. Most researchers will have published journal articles or an abbreviated form of the work in the RCN Research Series. You may need to refer to the original work if you are unclear about the results or methodology and wish to clarify these before thinking about implementing the findings.

Glossary

abstract   (page 13) (at the beginning of a research report or thesis) A summary of why the study was done and the main results.

abstracting journal   (page 15) A publication that summarizes published material in a particular subject area.

action research   (page 37) A method of undertaking social research that incorporates the researcher's involvement as a direct and deliberate part of the research, i.e. the researcher acts as a change agent.

appendices   (page 67) The purpose of the appendices is to expand on information that was only mentioned briefly in the report, e.g. instructions to subjects, questionnaires, interview or observation schedules.

bias   (page 48) Any tendency for results to differ from the true value in some consistent way. This could be due to experimenter bias (lack of objectivity), sample bias (non-random sample) or statistical bias (within the statistical analysis chosen).

bibliographic software   (page 20) A commercial computer disk that is supplied with templates that allow the storage, cross-referencing and retrieval of references, abstracts and notes. Some disks will also format references into various styles for printing.

bibliography   (page 67) List of material that has been read and informs the study but has not been referred to within the text.

British Nursing Index (BNI)   (page 15) A database incorporating the RCN Nursing Bibliography, RCN Nurse ROM and the Nursing and Midwifery Index. Includes over 220 health-related journals, with 9000 references being added each year. Produced for the Internet, on CD-ROM and in printed form.

CD-ROM   (page 12) A computer disk imprinted with information that can be accessed and read but information cannot be added.

Chi-squared (χ^2)   (page 61) A statistical test based on the frequencies with which events occur. It demonstrates the expected distribution of the sum of squares for scores according to the normal curve (bell shaped).

CINAHL   (page 13) Cumulative Index to Nursing and Allied Health Literature, a CD-ROM.

coefficient of correlation   (page 63) A numerical index used to indicate the degree of correspondence (match) between two sets of measurements.

construct validity   (page 48) Refers to whether the research tool forms an accurate assessment of the theoretical construct that it is supposed to measure. Does it accurately reflect the theory underlying the idea?

control group   (page 40) A group of subjects (people or things) who, in the course of an experimental research project, do not experience the factor under consideration, so that a comparison can be made with the effects produced on the experimental group (see below).

criterion validity   (page 48) When validity is assessed by measuring it against some external criterion, e.g. comparing nursing exam results with IQ scores.

cross-sectional study   (page 39) Involves the comparison of two or more groups at one point in time.

data   (page 12) Information, facts.

database   (page 12) A source that contains information or facts.

degrees of freedom (df)   (page 61) Associated with sampling distribution and is calculated as part of a test of significance.

dependent variable   (in experimental research) (page 40). The aspect being studied to see whether the experimental factor, the independent variable (see below), has had any effect.

descriptive research, design   (page 37) Research that aims to provide a knowledge base when little is known of a phenomenon or to clarify a situation or describe subject characteristics, e.g. surveys, case studies, grounded theory.

distribution   (page 63) The relative frequencies with which scores of different size occur. *See* standard deviation.

ethics   (page 37) The philosophical study of the moral value of human conduct and of the rules and principles that ought to govern it.

ethnography   (page 43) A qualitative research approach developed by anthropologists with the purpose of describing an aspect of culture, but is also aimed at learning about the culture or factor being studied.

evidence-based practice   (page 1) Systematically appraising clinical situations and then using up-to-date research findings as a basis for nursing decisions.

experimental group   (page 40) A group of subjects (people or things) who, in the course of an experimental research project, are caused to experience the factor under consideration.

experimental research   (page 37) Research that tests a hypothesis by means of controlled manipulation of variables.

hardware   (page 20) Equipment used in a computer system such as the central processing unit, peripheral devices and memory.

hypothesis   (page 34) A statement based on knowledge or information that has yet to be proved or disproved.

implementation   (page 71) Carrying out or putting into action.

independent variable   (in experimental research) (page 40). The experimental factor which is deliberately manipulated, given to the experimental group and not the control group.

information technology   (page 12) The technology of the production, storage and communication of information using computers and microelectronics.

internal consistency   (page 47) A measure of reliability in which separate items in a test are correlated with the total scores for the test.

interscorer/interjudge reliability   (page 47) A test of reliability when subjective judgements are involved in an assessment situation. The scores from two independent raters are correlated to look for agreement between them.

interview   (page 39) A formal discussion between two people usually for a specific purpose.

key words   (page 10) Significant words used to describe the content of a document, chapter or idea.

level of significance   (page 61) The probability of rejecting the null hypothesis when the result of statistical tests of significance is, for example, 0.05 or lower (5% level of significance). *See* statistical significance and statistical inference.

literature review   (page 33) A brief résumé of previous and related work.

longitudinal study   (page 39) A group of people are studied over time in order to follow any development or change in a dependent variable.

mean   (page 54) The arithmetic average.

median   (page 54) The number that occurs in the middle of an ordered sequence of scores.

MEDLINE   (page 13) Computer database that covers over 3700 journals and 8 million references, mainly from the USA.

method/methodology   (page 37) The way in which the researcher has tried to fulfil the aim of the study. Methodology includes such aspects as the type of research employed, sample size and selection, research tools used and ways of collecting and analysing data.

mode   (page 54) The score that occurs most frequently in a set of scores.

non-participant observation   (page 46) When the observer is not part of the situation being observed.

null hypothesis   (page 34) This states that there will be no difference in the dependent variable between the control and experimental groups (i.e. that the experiment will not work). The null hypothesis will be discarded if the experimental hypothesis is supported.

observations   (page 39) *See* participant observation and non-participant observation.

participant observation   (page 46) When an observer takes part in a situation that is being observed.

phenomenology   (page 43) A method of inquiry that looks at what life experiences are like for people.

pilot study   (page 46) A preliminary study carried out to test the proposed method and research tools for the main study.

population   (page 43) The total number of people or things which could be treated as subjects in a research project.

probability *(P)*   (page 60) The likelihood of an event occurring by chance, rather than being caused by the experimental variables. *P* is expressed numerically on a scale from 0 to 1.

qualitative research   (page 38) Research which paints a picture in words and aims to identify concepts and common themes.

quantitative research   (page 38) Research in which the data is numerical and seeks to test hypotheses by statistical analysis of the data.

questionnaire   (page 39) A written list of questions. They come in various forms from the open ended, such as 'what do you think about', to the forced choice, where the respondents can only answer yes or no to the question.

randomized controlled trial   (page 41) An experimental design characterized by the manipulation of the independent variable, random assignment of individual subjects to the conditions and all other factors being controlled.

random sampling   (page 44) The systematic selection of a sample to ensure that all members of a population stand an equal chance of being selected.

references   (page 67) The listing of books and journals that have been cited in the text.

reliability   (page 47) (of a test) Whether or not the same test will give the same results when used under the same conditions on different occasions.

research-based profession   (page 1) When nursing uses research methods and research findings to assess, plan, implement and evaluate nursing care. Research informs problem-solving, decision-making and all aspects of nursing.

research design   (page 37) The selection of the most appropriate method of inquiry that will answer the research questions and aim of the study. May be qualitative or quantitative, descriptive, experimental or action research.

research tools   (page 37) Tools used to carry out research, e.g. questionnaires, audio and video recording, interview schedules, observations (either behavioural or physiological, participant or non-participant).

sample   (page 37) A selection of people or things from the possible population (see above) to be subjects for a research study.

semi-structured interview   (page 50) When there is some framework to the discussion but rather in the form of subject headings rather than precise questions.

software   (page 20) Computer programs as opposed to the computer itself.

standard deviation   (page 62) A measure of distribution, calculated from the amount by which each score differs from the mean of all scores.

statistical inference   (page 61) Drawn from the testing of data for level of significance. In other words, whether it is likely that the results obtained were due to chance or due to the independent variable. *See* level of significance and statistical significance.

statistical significance   (page 60) A conclusion that the results achieved have little probability of occurring by chance alone. If the result is statistically significant, e.g. below the 0.05 level (1 in 20), then we can be fairly confident that something other than chance produced the result.

structured interview   (page 50) When the discussion is carried out in a very precise manner, addressing the same issues in the same way for all participants, rather like a verbal questionnaire.

subjects   (page 40) People, animals or things that form the sample in research.

synonym   (page 10) A word that means the same or nearly the same as another word.

temporal stability   (page 47) When a research tool has been tested for reliability using the test–retest method. In other words, when the tool is given to a group of people on two occasions, the scores on the first occasion correlate with the scores on the second occasion.

tests of significance   (page 61) Tests indicating whether the difference between the observed result and those expected from the original hypothesis are likely to be due to chance.

t-test   (page 62) A test of significance that is distribution dependent.

unstructured or open interview   (page 50) When there is no format or framework from which to carry out the interview; only the subject of the discussion is stated.

validity   (page 47) (of a test) Whether or not the test measures what it is supposed to measure.

variable   (page 40) An attribute, quality or characteristic that can be varied, observed and measured. *See* dependent and independent variables.

web site   (page 15) Pages of graphically presented material on the Internet.